Developing Successful
Health Care Education
Simulation Centers

The Consortium Model

About the Authors

Pamela R. Jeffries, PhD, RN, FAAN, ANEF, is nationally known for her research and work in developing simulations and online teaching and learning. At the Johns Hopkins University School of Nursing and throughout the academic community, she is well regarded for her expertise in experiential learning, innovative teaching strategies, new pedagogies, and the delivery of content using technology in nursing education. Dr. Jeffries served as the project director for a national simulation study funded by the National League for Nursing (NLN) and the Laerdal Corporation. She was named to the same role for a second NLN and Laerdal grant to facilitate the development of web-based courses for faculty development in simulation and a national simulation innovation resource center. She is now serving on a 5-year Health Resources and Services Administration grant to develop Health Information Technology Scholars. She has previously been awarded several grants to support her research and is the recipient of several teaching awards, including the NLN Lucile Petry Leone Award. She has been a consultant on the Economic Opportunities for 2015 (EcO$_{15}$) consortium in southern Indiana, serving as the simulation specialist and assisting with overall faculty development, goal setting, and strategic planning.

Jim Battin, BS, is the president of Strategic Consulting Group, Inc., located in Columbus, Indiana. He started the company in 1998 and has served clients in private and public sectors. Strategic Consulting Group, Inc., specializes in strategic planning and project management of projects involving multiple partners in large-scale initiatives. Most recently, he has led the development of a health care consortium made up of health care partners throughout 10 counties in introducing simulation technology in nursing education programs in education and clinical settings.

Prior to the start-up of Strategic Consulting Group, Mr. Battin completed a 25-year career at Cummins, Inc., primarily in the area of human resources (HR) and total quality systems. While at Cummins, he had responsibility to develop an HR audit system for manufacturing plants worldwide and implemented training and continuous improvement programs to increase the effectiveness of HR processes and systems. He has a bachelor's degree in psychology from Purdue University and completed graduate studies in organizational psychology.

Developing Successful Health Care Education Simulation Centers

The Consortium Model

Pamela R. Jeffries, PhD, RN, FAAN, ANEF

Jim Battin, BS

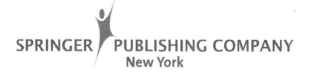

SPRINGER PUBLISHING COMPANY
New York

Springer Publishing Company, LLC
11 West 42nd Street
New York, NY 10036
www.springerpub.com

Acquisitions Editor: Margaret Zuccarini
Composition: diacriTech

ISBN: 978-0-8261-2954-3
E-book ISBN: 978-0-8261-2955-0

12 13 14/ 5 4 3 2

The author and the publisher of this work have made every effort to use sources believed to be reliable to provide information that is accurate and compatible with the standards generally accepted at the time of publication. Because medical science is continually advancing, our knowledge base continues to expand. Therefore, as new information becomes available, changes in procedures become necessary. We recommend that the reader always consult current research and specific institutional policies before performing any clinical procedure. The author and publisher shall not be liable for any special, consequential, or exemplary damages resulting, in whole or in part, from the readers' use of, or reliance on, the information contained in this book. The publisher has no responsibility for the persistence or accuracy of URLs for external or third-party Internet Web sites referred to in this publication and does not guarantee that any content on such Web sites is, or will remain, accurate or appropriate.

CIP data available from the Library of Congress

Special discounts on bulk quantities of our books are available to corporations, professional associations, pharmaceutical companies, health care organizations, and other qualifying groups.
If you are interested in a custom book, including chapters from more than one of our titles, we can provide that service as well.

For details, please contact:
Special Sales Department, Springer Publishing Company, LLC
11 West 42nd Street, 15th Floor, New York, NY 10036-8002
Phone: 877-687-7476 or 212-431-4370; Fax: 212-941-7842
Email: sales@springerpub.com

Printed in the United States of America by Gasch Printing.

We dedicate this book to simulation user groups

who are considering or implementing the development of

regional, state, or national consortia.

Our vision is that we will continuously learn from each other

and improve patient safety and quality care

through the use of clinical simulation education methodology.

Contents

List of Contributors

Mary Lou Brunell
Florida Center for Nursing

Bonnie Driggers
Oregon Simulation Alliance

Scott A. Engum
Fairbanks Simulation Center

Dave Galle
Southeast Indiana Health Care Consortium

Paula Gubrud-Howe
Oregon Consortium for Nursing Education

Debi Sampsel
Nursing Institute of West Central Ohio

Michael Seropian
Oregon Simulation Alliance

KT Waxman
Bay Area Simulation Collaborative

Simulation Consortia and Leaders

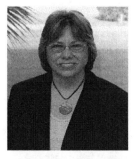

Mary Lou Brunell

Florida Center for Nursing
The Quality and Unity in Nursing (QUIN) Council was formally established in June 1990 with the mission to promote quality and unity for nurses and nursing in Florida. Members include state-level organizations led by nurses that have a mission and purpose consistent with the mission and objectives of QUIN Council. Through collaborative effort under the leadership of QUIN Council, the Florida Center for Nursing (Center) was established in statute (FS 464.0195) by the 2001 Florida Legislature with three primary goals:

1. Develop a strategic statewide plan for nursing manpower in this state
2. Convene various groups representative of nurses, other health care providers, business and industry, consumers, legislators, and educators
3. Enhance and promote recognition, reward, and renewal activities for nurses in the state

The Center described the need for a two-prong approach to resolve Florida's nursing shortage: (1) maximize the production of new nurses through education and (2) increase retention of the existing nurse workforce. In 2009, the executive director of the Center asked The Blue Foundation for a Healthy Florida (TBF) to partner with them in an effort to promote the use of simulation technology in Florida nurse education. TBF received a Partners Investing in Nursing's Future grant and contracted with the Center to conduct the project with the goal of maximizing the use of simulation technology in the preparation of new nurses and continuing education of current registered nurses in Florida, thus addressing the nursing shortage by increasing the nurse supply through increased production and retention. An advisory panel provides oversight and direction to the project with representation from the simulation industry, all levels of nursing education programs, the hospital industry, and existing simulation centers.

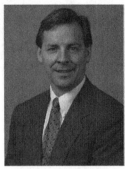

Scott A. Engum

The Simulation Center at Fairbanks Hall, Indiana University School of Nursing
The Simulation Center at Fairbanks Hall is a collaborative effort of Indiana University Health and Indiana University Schools of Medicine and Nursing. The center is 30,000 square feet and is divided into four main areas that include Acute Care, Virtual Hospital, Virtual Clinic, and Skills Area. The rooms within the Acute Care area include an operating room, emergency room, intensive care unit, ambulance, and multipurpose space. The Virtual Hospital houses five inpatient rooms and a neonatal/obstetrical suite. The Virtual Clinic has 10 outpatient exam rooms, and the Skills Area is divided into two large rooms.

The center is staffed by 15 employees and over 30 standardized patients that support education. The center has been very fortunate that all three partners continue to work collaboratively whenever possible to create an interprofessional atmosphere and realistic setting. The center has been open since August 2009 and continues to expand its customer base and support staff. The three partners contribute an educational liaison that assists in curricular development, and these individuals have been instrumental in driving collaborative initiatives. In addition to providing medical and nursing students curricular opportunities, as well as hospital-based orientation programs, the postgraduate residency programs have begun transitioning a number of educational opportunities to the simulation center.

The Simulation Center at Fairbanks Hall was built not just to enhance medical education on the Indiana University campus, but to become a regional and state resource tool. Area hospital systems and the regional campuses of the School of Medicine utilize the simulation center to meet curricular needs.

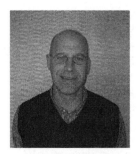

Dave Galle

Southeast Indiana Health Care Consortium
The Southeast Indiana Health Care Consortium was formed in 2008 as part of a regional grant and program called Economic Opportunities for 2015 (EcO_{15}). The region consists of 10 counties in a predominantly rural section of Indiana.

The vision of the EcO_{15} health care initiative is to improve the quality of health care education in Southeast Indiana to provide the quality and quantity of health care professionals in the region to assure patient safety and outcomes for its citizens.

Members of the health care consortium include representatives from secondary education, five postsecondary institutions, seven hospitals, Area Health Education Center, and the Community Education Coalition, a 501C3 organization.

The three main goals of the health care consortium are as follows: (1) develop the infrastructure for the use of simulation methodology in the education system, (2) increase the capacity of nursing graduates in the region, and (3) provide coordination through the development of a regional health care network of partners.

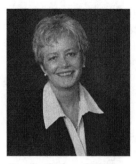

Paula Gubrud-Howe

Simulation and Clinical Learning Center at the Oregon Health and Science University (OHSU) and the Oregon Consortium for Nursing Education (OCNE)

The Oregon Consortium for Nursing Education (OCNE) is a statewide coalition established to find a long-term solution to the looming nursing shortage and to reform nursing curriculum so that tomorrow's nurses can better serve Oregon's aging and increasingly diverse population. OCNE seeks to increase capacity in schools of nursing by making the best use of scarce faculty, classrooms, and clinical training resources in the delivery of a shared curriculum on 13 campuses, including 8 community colleges and the 5 campuses of the Oregon Health & Science University (OHSU) School of Nursing. Community college students are coadmitted to their home community college and OHSU. The partnership's shared admission criteria, courses, and progression policies facilitate seamless progression in the curriculum, allowing associate-degree students to pursue baccalaureate nursing education in their home community.

The innovative competency-based curriculum was designed through the collaborative efforts involving faculty from all partner schools and focuses on health promotion, chronic illness care, end-of-life care, and prevalent conditions in acute care. Population-based health and leadership are introduced early in the curriculum and spiraled throughout all course work. Through partnership with health care systems, the OCNE partners have developed a transformational model for clinical education that is currently in the early phase of implementation. The National League for Nursing (NLN), the Carnegie Foundation for the Advancement of Teaching (through its Study on Preparation of the Professions), and the Institute of Medicine Future of Nursing report have endorsed OCNE as a national model for nursing education reform.

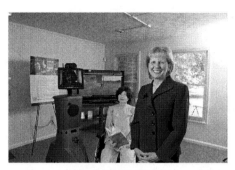

Debi Sampsel

Nursing Institute of West Central Ohio

Leaders from nursing education programs and health care organizations in 2004 formed the Nursing Institute of West Central Ohio to address shifts in the nursing workforce facing the region and the rest of the nation. The Nursing Institute is supported primarily by its "Sustainability Partners" Premier Health Partners, Sinclair Community College, Wright State University, and Graceworks Lutheran Services. This 22-county collaborative venture among programs of nursing, health care organizations, public health, businesses, the military, and the local Veterans Administration acts as a catalyst through which the latest technologies and best practices in nursing and nursing education can be tested, demonstrated, and spread rapidly into real-world situations. The Nursing Institute continues to address shifts in the nursing workforce such as the rising average age of nurses by exploring methods of recruiting, educating, and retaining new nurses as well as expanding educational program capacities by better utilizing the teaching skills of experienced nurses.

One of the ways the Nursing Institute, headquartered at Wright State University, and its many partners are advancing the nursing profession's knowledge, research, and practice is through the use of various types of simulation. The Nursing Institute's flagship simulation facility is located in a residential home, called the Living Laboratory Smart Technology House. The house is purposefully designed to maximize various forms of simulation. One of the most interesting deployments of simulation scenarios is through the use of simulators to create an 11-member intergenerational family. The "Techy" family resides in this home that is situated on Bethany Village Campus, which is a 100-acre continuing care retirement campus. The home-like atmosphere creates the perfect setting for the transformation of nursing into a future focused community-based delivery model. The outcomes derived from the work in the Living Laboratory are shared with the entire collaborative group. The various organizational collaborators participate at different levels of engagement with simulation and the other available technology.

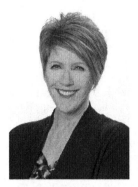

KT Waxman

The Bay Area Simulation Collaborative (BASC)
The Bay Area Simulation Collaborative (BASC) is a 600-member academic/service partnership created through grant funding from the Gordon and Betty Moore Foundation to develop a common language for simulation, train faculty, write and share scenarios, and conduct research. The goal of this project is to enhance the quality and skills of students and staff nurses and share information and best practice.

The BASC is comprised of representatives from schools of nursing and hospitals in the 11 San Francisco Bay Area counties, which is governed by an operating and advisory committee. The California Institute for Nursing & Health Care (CINHC) provides leadership for the BASC. The project involves faculty development for nursing faculty and hospital educators in the Bay Area over a 3-year period. Four levels of training have been developed beginning with basic fundamentals through a train-the-trainer model. Faculty development is integral to incorporating the use of simulation in nurse education curriculum.

To date, almost 1,000 faculty and nurse educators have received simulation education through the BASC with our standardized curriculum. By utilizing simulation in schools, hospitals, and regional centers, we hope to enhance the nurses' competencies and confidence, which will result in increased safety for the patients we serve.

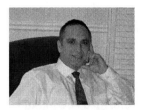

Michael Seropian

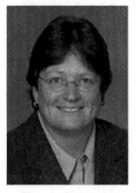

Bonnie Driggers

Oregon Simulation Alliance
First established in 2003, the Oregon Simulation Alliance (OSA) is a unique public-private, multisector, multidisciplinary, not-for-profit organization (501(c)3) whose vision and mission are the following:

VISION: The OSA envisions an efficient statewide network established for the application of innovative technology resources, information and training systems for existing and future healthcare professionals.

MISSION: To ensure quality patient care for all Oregonians through the use of simulation technology and practice to help healthcare workers to be more confident, competent and compassionate in providing patient care.

(http://oregonsimulation.com/about/vision-mission-and-history/)

The OSA is an independent organization, with formal bylaws, policies, and procedures, that uses a subscription model to help increase capacity of competent simulation-based education providers/instructors in Oregon. Subscribers come from both academia and service. The ultimate goal is for simulation instructors and programs to address the quality and safety needs of the health care workforce at the pre- and post-licensure level across disciplines. This includes student development, ongoing provider competency development, provider remediation, and maintenance of certification. In order to fulfill its mission and vision, the OSA has provided a variety of services, including but not limited to:

- Simulation instructor courses for novice to advanced beginners.
- Access to simulation equipment pricing agreements with a variety of vendors.
- Apprentice opportunities for simulation educators.
- Training for simulation technicians.
- Access to specialized education in debriefing.
- Statewide simulation networking conferences highlighting local and national simulation educators.
- Access to new equipment demonstrations.
- Advice and mentoring to simulation programs regarding program development.

The OSA's approach has been unique in that it has used a market-based strategy. Its focus changes with the market need within the state. This flexibility has allowed it to shift from an initial focus on nursing to its current focus on first responders. The Board of the OSA is made up of volunteer physicians, nurses, and individuals from allied health. The work of the OSA is coordinated by a paid Executive Director. The OSA's implementation model and strategy have been implemented and modified by many other groups in the United States and internationally.

Foreword

Simulation in health care is still in its infancy. Most of us in simulation-based education began our careers as practitioners, educators, or both. Many educators who want to start a simulation-based education program may not know where to begin because they often lack business, project planning, and simulation expertise. In this setting we have seen the emergence of simulation collaborations across the globe. Simulation by its very nature is multiprofessional, which has likely contributed to the natural migration to a collaborative use model. The simulation community is in need of a road map to develop collaborations effectively in simulation. This book will serve as an important resource for those who are beginning collaborations in simulation, regardless of discipline or domain. It should also be viewed as a point of reference for evaluating existing collaborations.

We have had the opportunity over the last 8 years to participate in or guide the development of many collaborations around simulation. Some have been small and local, while others have been at a state and national level. The content and exemplars in this book do support many of the core principles readers should consider as they implement a collaborative simulation model. Many existing collaborations have been formed around a purchase of equipment or funding from a grant or foundation without a specific plan for the collaboration, its educational purpose, governance, or sustainability. Many collaborations struggle without this level of specificity when initial funds are depleted or when economic times are difficult.

Starting with clarification of purpose or goal is important. Frye's Levels of Collaboration, for example, help partners decide how they want or are able to collaborate given their specific circumstances and geopolitical environments. Some, like in Idaho, have initially developed as "networks" where they share a common goal and, by Frye's Levels of Collaboration definition, are still loosely defined yet are still considered as an organized entity. Many will start at this point and evolve, much as we have seen in California and other regions around the world. Others are more organized and formally collaborative, in that they share resources, ideas, and decision making and have frequent and prioritized communications, such as the Oregon Consortium for Nursing Education or the Oregon Simulation Alliance.

We would like to encourage readers to carefully analyze the principles of strategic planning, partnership development, and collaboration in simulation outlined in this book. This book will help developing as well as existing programs as readers reflect upon their programs and improve them so that educators and administrators are free to focus their attention on teaching and learning through simulation.

We encourage the readers to apply what they have learned after reading the book and then go back and read it again, learn more, and apply more of your learning.

Bonnie Driggers, MS, MPA, RN
Michael Seropian, MD, FRCPC

Preface

Today's nurse graduates enter a changing health care environment that includes high-acuity patients, rapid patient turnover, sophisticated technological environments, and staffing shortages. New nurses arrive on the floor with little hands-on experience, woefully underprepared for a fast-paced profession that demands the ability to critically assess and respond to complex situations with flexibility and precision. Education that leverages simulation technology can help educational and clinical facilities provide practical education and experience to nursing students and professionals safely and efficiently.

Simulation exercises have enjoyed a long history in nursing education. Whether the student practices intramuscular and subcutaneous injections on an orange, or cardiopulmonary resuscitation on a manikin, the exercises deploy "a research or teaching technique that," according to the Encyclopedia Britannica (2008), "reproduces actual events and processes under test conditions" to transmit knowledge. Rather than didactic learning, this type of experiential learning actively engages the learner in gaining knowledge through firsthand and visceral education. Technological advances have enabled increasingly complex simulation exercises that allow novices to practice new skills and experience uncommon or risky nursing challenges with supervision and feedback. Unfortunately, simulation laboratories do not come cheap: Depending upon its size and complexity, developing one can run well into six figures.

How can nursing education and clinical facilities make simulation education available to large numbers of student nurses and professionals in an efficient, cost-effective manner? Through a nursing simulation consortium.

Although simulation technology continues to gain favor and applicability, the literature detailing the consortium-building process remains lacking. We hope that our simulation consortium model can help. The model steps hospital administrators, nurse educators, or grant managers through the process of creating a consortium to share brainpower and resources for simulation education.

BOOK STRUCTURE AND FORMAT

Written for academics, hospital administrators, nurse educators, and others interested in sharing simulation resources to better prepare nurses and nursing students for safe, evidence-based practice, this book provides a model for consortium-building, from early brainstorming to best sustainability practices.

The use of technology for nursing simulation education is still in its infancy, and there is no "right" way to go about this work. However, we can share the ideas, strategies, and processes that worked for us, based on our experiences as a simulation expert and organizational strategy development consultant. Chapter 1 contextualizes the need for a simulation consortium, citing contributing workplace and economic factors, while Chapters 2 through 11 follow the model through a series of 11 steps, from building a consortium to ensuring sustainability. A brief description of each chapter or model element follows:

Chapter 1: Why Build a Simulation Consortium?
This chapter explores the current practice needs of nursing education; the value of simulation technology for one organization is complicated by logistical and financial considerations.

- A simulation consortium allows stakeholders in nursing education to share knowledge, financial and educational resources, and ideas to train large numbers of nursing students and professionals, as well as provide training for simulation educators.

Chapter 2: Consortium Development
- Building the founding network
- Establishing the vision and purpose of the consortium
- Developing early leadership
- Collecting information
- Organizing a growing leadership

Chapter 3: Consortium Leadership and Management
- Developing a governance structure, including committees and task forces, and detailing roles and responsibilities
- Establishing a process for communicating and sharing information among consortium members
- Integrating the principles of stewardship

Chapter 4: Collaboration
- Developing relationships to form and evolve the consortium
- Establishing goals through cooperation

Chapter 5: Strategy Development
- Identifying the consortium's important principles and goals
- Prioritizing the consortium's efforts
- Establishing a process to track the consortium's progress
- Developing a data collection process
- Formulating strategies, goals, activity, and resource requirements

Chapter 6: Strategy Evaluation
- Using the simulation strategy evaluation tool to reinforce achievement of the consortium's strategies

Chapter 7: Professional Development
- Defining the knowledge, skills, abilities, training, and education required of the consortium, educators, staff members, and partners throughout the region
- Creating a professional development plan in support of the strategic plan, goals, and objectives

Chapter 8: Strategy Implementation
- Planning, organizing, directing, monitoring outcomes, and reflecting on lessons learned to develop more accurate planning, more effective organizing, greater efficiency, and better outcomes
- Building confidence in the consortium's effectiveness
- Implementing continuous improvement

Chapter 9: Reflection and Renewal
- Reviewing results of strategic plan outcomes and the strategy evaluation
- Developing momentum and instituting change in support of the next planning cycle
- Building trust, developing common expectations, learning, and grounding the level of collective commitment to the consortium's vision and mission

Chapter 10: Sustainability
- Securing long-term funding
- Progressing to the next planning cycle with excitement and cooperation

Chapter 11: Simulation Consortium Model Review
- Completing the system loop
- Reinventing the consortium as appropriate, with lessons learned from the process

The model represents the typical flow of the consortium process, but as you will see from our examples, the structure provides ample room for variation. Each chapter concludes with a section titled "Lessons Learned," which details the valuable educational points that we and our consortium colleagues picked up along the way—and could have used to make our work that much easier, had we known them earlier.

We have also interspersed the text with illustrative examples from leaders from six simulation consortia across the United States. (For information about each of these consortia, please see pp. xiii–xx.) These consortia range in size, geographical location and range, and capacity, and they have assembled for varying reasons, built different governing structures, and approached their strategic plans from various angles. They share in common, however, a firm belief that collaboration inspires innovation, and that the future of simulation in nursing education is without limits. We thank each of these health care leaders for their input: Mary Lou Brunell, Scott A. Engum, Dave Galle, Paula Gubrud-Howe, Debi Sampsel, KT Waxman, Michael Seropian, and Bonnie Driggers. This book owes much to their ideas, encouragement, and support for the collaborative process. (To learn more about their consortium work, see the following pages.)

Pamela R. Jeffries, PhD, RN, FAAN, ANEF
Jim Battin, BS

Acknowledgments

Our sincere appreciation goes out to the following contributors who provided insights and lessons learned from their experiences in simulation center start-ups and the development of regional and state consortia.

- Mary Lou Brunell, Executive Director of the Florida Center for Nursing
- Scott A. Engum, Director of the Simulation Center at Fairbanks Hall at Indiana University School of Medicine
- Dave Galle, Executive Director of the Community Education Coalition in Columbus, Indiana
- Paula Gubrud-Howe, Assistant Professor of the Oregon Health and Science University School of Nursing
- Debi Sampsel, Executive Director of the Nursing Institute of West Central Ohio
- KT Waxman, Program Director, Bay Area Simulation Collaborative; California Institute for Nursing & Health Care
- Michael Seropian and Bonnie Driggers, Oregon Simulation Alliance

Their stories provided us with affirmation that the simulation center consortium model we are presenting in this book is consistent with their experiences. In addition, they provided insights and lessons learned that are invaluable to those readers who are sorting through the opportunities and challenges that are presented in regional and statewide consortium development. Thank you for sharing your experiences and promising practices with us all.

The Southeast Indiana Health Care Consortium experience provided both of us the opportunity to experience and document the steps presented in this book that include the planning, implementation, and sustainability of a regional consortium start-up. We thank John Burnett, Chief Executive Officer of the Community Education, located in Columbus, Indiana, and Sherry Stark, President and CEO, Heritage Fund, the Community Foundation of Bartholomew

County, Indiana, and Lilly Endowment Inc., whose generosity made the Economic Opportunities for 2015 (EcO$_{15}$) health care initiative a reality. We also want to acknowledge the EcO$_{15}$ Health Care Steering Committee and Simulation Task Force members who provided leadership and direction for the simulation center initiative.

Special thanks go to Cathleen Nielan, freelance editor from Baltimore, Maryland, who took concepts and turned them into more concrete action steps that more accurately describe the pathway from planning to implementation of a simulation center consortium. Her questions pushed our thinking and helped us produce a better product of our work.

Margaret Zuccarini, Christina Ferraro, and the editorial team at Springer Publishing Company provided us direction and support in the development of the manuscript and the flow of content in the book. Their assistance is greatly appreciated.

We would like to thank our families for their continued love, support, patience, and encouragement throughout this undertaking. They gave up their time with us to provide us the opportunity to contribute to the advancement of simulation education for educators and students, which will ultimately benefit and improve patient safety and the overall quality of health care for all of us.

P.R.J.
J.L.B.

ONE

Why Develop a Consortium for Simulation Educators?

Never before in history has innovation offered promise of so much to so many in so short a time.
　—Bill Gates

*A*s hospital administrative leaders, you have noticed the great dis-
connect between the academic preparation of nursing students
and the needs and expectations of your organizations. You have also
seen the price in time, management, efficiency, and patient safety:
Inexperience costs, every time. As health care becomes increasingly
complex, with rapid technological advances, more patient traffic,
and greater demands on health care professionals, you need nurse
graduates who can hit the floor running—those who can critically
assess and respond to complicated, charged situations with confidence in their practice. Unfortunately, many schools of nursing are
not turning such graduates out. Why is this the case, and how can a
consortium of simulation educators close that gap?

Both academic and administrative leaders agree on the value
of clinical simulation in health care education, yet the expense of a
high-fidelity simulation center prohibits many organizations from
embarking upon this effort. The solution? A consortium. Defined
by Merriam-Webster's Dictionary as "an agreement, combination,
or group (as of companies) formed to undertake an enterprise
beyond the resources of any one member," a consortium—regional,
statewide, or national—allows nursing education institutions, clinical agencies, and health care organizations to share resources in preparing health care professionals for quality, safe patient care.

The background for this state of affairs is complicated, involving changes in the nursing profession, economic demands, and a
changing student demographic. However, through the collaborative
work of a regional, state, or national consortium, health care organizations can provide hands-on, visceral learning experiences—like

those offered by simulation education—to train large numbers of nursing students and professionals in a low-risk, controlled environment.

THE PRACTICE–PREPARATION GAP

You have seen nursing graduates fumble at the bedside, or panic in a critical situation. Unfortunately, your experience is not singular—this gap between preparation and practice is widespread. In 2008, the Nursing Executive Center of the Advisory Board Company surveyed nursing school academic leaders and frontline hospital administrators and identified six areas of concern for hospital leaders regarding the practice readiness of recent nurse graduates (Berkow, Virkstis, Stewart, & Conway, 2009). According to the survey, almost 90% of nursing school leaders stated that new graduates were prepared in these areas, whereas *only 10% of nurse administrators believe that recent nurse graduates have the practical skills and knowledge to do their jobs* (see Exhibit 1.1).

EXHIBIT 1.1
"Practice Readiness": Areas of Concern for Hospital Leaders

1. Clinical knowledge
2. Technical skills
3. Critical thinking
4. Communications
5. Professionalism
6. Management of responsibilities

In response to statistics like these, national organizations such as the National League for Nursing and the American Association of Colleges of Nursing have challenged nurse educators to develop new clinical redesign models to better prepare future nurses for clinical practice, promoting safe, quality patient care while accommodating such changes in the health care profession as employment growth and increasing emphasis on interdisciplinary teamwork.

NURSING SHORTAGES

The American Association of Colleges of Nursing projects a national "nursing shortage that is expected to intensify as baby boomers age and the need for health care grows"—a problem further complicated by "the fact that nursing colleges and universities across the country are struggling to expand enrollment levels to meet the rising demand for nursing care." As the median age of registered nurses continues to increase, not enough younger workers are replacing them. As a result, employers in some parts of the country are reporting difficulties in attracting and retaining nurses.

All of the consortia interviewed for this book cited nursing shortages as one of the reasons for their development. With fewer nurses shouldering more responsibilities, health care organizations struggle to increase worker efficiency in a safe environment.

AN EXPANDING JOB MARKET

Health care organizations need to prepare for an influx of new health care professionals. According to the U.S. Bureau of Labor Statistics (2010a, 2010b), health care is one of the largest industries in the United States economy, providing 14.3 million jobs in 2008. Employment will continue to grow because of the following factors:

1. The proportion of the population in older age groups—which have a higher incidence of injury—will grow faster than the total population between 2008 and 2018. The number of people aged 65 years and more is projected to increase from 39 million in 2010 to 69 million in 2030. About 20% of the total population will be older than 65 years in 2030, compared with the current 13%.
2. Advances in medical technology will continue to improve the survival rate of severely ill and injured patients, who will then need extensive therapy and care.

3. Improvements in diagnostic tests and surgical procedures, along with patient desires to be treated at home, will cause a shift from inpatient to less-expensive outpatient and home care.

Furthermore, 10 of the 20 fastest growing occupations are related to health care, including home health aides, personal and home care aides, medical assistants, pharmacy technicians, dental hygienists, physical therapists, physical therapist assistants or aides, and physician assistants.

Because of this employment growth, as well as expected turnover, health care workers at all levels of education and training will continue to be in demand. With health care as one of the few professional areas to see growth during a stagnant economy, our organizations must prepare to educate large numbers of new students and transitioning professionals.

INTERDISCIPLINARY WORK TRENDING UP

Since the publication of its reports, "Crossing the quality chasm" and "To err is human" in 2001, the Institute of Medicine has continued to emphasize interdisciplinary education, founded on quality improvement and informatics, as a better way to prepare health care professionals for practice. As this trend continues, health care education will need to implement ways in which different professions can collaborate and share resources. With the increased number of students enrolled in health care professional programs, combined with ethical imperatives for learning and reduced access to quality clinical experiences, medical and nursing education increasingly rely on simulations and simulated patients, particularly in interdisciplinary patient safety initiatives (Cleland, Abe, & Rethans, 2009).

SIMULATION EDUCATION CAN HELP

Simulation technology enables educators to meet these challenges by increasing knowledge and skills that can be transferred into clinical settings. Simulated environments and experiences allow instructors to create realistic clinical situations and observe student–patient communication, as well as student skills and clinical decision making, in a controlled environment. They can design simulations that focus on the following:

- Specific critical clinical activities, assessments, or interventions that require quick assessment and good clinical diagnostic skills
- Clinical situations that all students need to experience, but that are difficult for all to encounter on the clinical unit during a semester practicum
- Problem-solving encounters that require students to perform real-time assessments and clinical problem interventions

Through such high-fidelity simulations, students can learn how to make decisions based on their classroom knowledge and laboratory experience. This type of simulated experience bridges the gap between academe and clinical practice. Integration of theory and practice in simulated environments replaces educational practice that too often teaches nursing content in "silos." In that separate-but-equal model, students learn didactic content in the classroom, while they develop skills in a laboratory course. Simulations, however, provide students an opportunity to synthesize and apply their knowledge and skills in a safe and nonthreatening environment.

Disadvantages to Individual Simulation Centers

Unfortunately, many organizations find the implementation of simulation education to be simply too expensive and too onerous to make the investment alone. Initial faculty resistance, the complexity of the undertaking, and the administrative and financial costs can overwhelm the resources of a single institution.

A Complex Undertaking

Establishing a simulation laboratory requires a vast skill set: research and analytical abilities, business acumen, educational expertise, technical capabilities, and simulation experience, to name a few. Organizations must consider renovation requirements and costs, the logistics of developing and implementing a skills training program for educators and students, technical support, and system maintenance.

Resistance From Health Professional Educators

Not all educators feel prepared to design and implement simulations in their courses; nor do they understand the great potential of adopting this educational method (Brill & Galloway, 2009). Some believe that students cannot obtain high-quality, realistic clinical experiences unless they care for "real" patients on an actual clinical unit. Organizations need to dedicate time and energy to challenging these misperceptions and training a workforce in novel educational approaches.

Costs

Simulation technology does not come cheap. In 2006, McIntosh, Macario, Flanagan, and Gaba identified start-up costs of $876,485 to rebuild existing facilities and buy equipment, with fixed costs of $361,425 per annum and variable costs of $311 per course hour. Pressure to control hospital administrative costs continues to grow, yet ignoring opportunities to increase learning and efficiency among health care professionals can jeopardize the financial welfare of health care providers.

Clearly, a single organization's investment in a simulation laboratory is significant among the many barriers to the use of simulation technology in nursing education. Establishing a simulation consortium of equally invested institutions allows you to share not only the financial investment but also the responsibilities and advantages of such a valuable educational venture.

THE POWER OF MANY: BENEFITS OF A CONSORTIUM

A simulation consortium establishes an academia–service partnership dedicated to helping health care institutions provide the benefits of simulation education to a wide range of users. Its collaborative opportunities include business models, funding, equipment, pedagogical training, faculty development, scenario building, and technological support.

THE SIMULATION CONSORTIUM MODEL

This book provides a simulation consortium model that uses a team approach, which incorporates the varied perspectives of different health care disciplines, toward interdisciplinary education and practice, which improves patient care while decreasing overall health care costs (Gardner, Chamberlain, Heestand, & Stowe, 2002). To successfully adopt this model, however, we must identify and consider its benefits and challenges, as outlined in Table 1.1.

Throughout the book, we use the simulation consortium model, with examples from various consortia, to show you how to leverage the benefits and minimize the challenges to achieve the expectations of all. As part of our research, we interviewed members of various county, urban, regional, and state consortia.

Although these consortia differ in size, scope, and needs, the simulation consortium model provides a systematic approach to plan, organize, and implement education simulation center programs. In particular, we were fortunate to discuss the origins and development of the first consortium of its kind, the Oregon Simulation Alliance (OSA), with Michael Seropian, MD, and Bonnie Driggers, MS, MPA, RN, experts in simulation education and two of the organization's founding members.

The Oregon Simulation Alliance: Exemplar Consortium

Many of the ideas and principles of the model presented here found their origins in the OSA. Established in 2003, the OSA provides resources and services to health care educators in service and academia, and across disciplines and sectors, for improving patient care through simulation methodologies and technologies.

TABLE 1.1
Benefits and Challenges of a Simulation Consortium

BENEFITS	CHALLENGES
• Delivering safer patient care	• No well-defined models for training students
• Respect and understanding of other team members	• Conflicting schedules
• Potential for shared resources in education and development	• Scheduling differences making co-learning a challenge
• Decreased costs to health care	• Different evaluation and expectations for clinical education
• Bridging the gap in health care education through multidisciplinary work	• Requirement of flexibility as interprofessional education is pursued
• Improved health care teams for patient care delivery	• New pedagogy

An independent, not-for-profit 501(c)(3) organization with an eye to sustainability, the OSA does not merely assist with funding; rather, it uses a market-based strategy to help health care networks across the state identify educational needs, tailor and implement simulation-based solutions, and ensure long-term growth. Since its beginning, the OSA has provided simulation consortia with a thoughtful, well considered model of collaborative development and sustainability.

According to Michael and Bonnie, this collaborative effort began with a gathering of individuals from a variety of organizations, including community colleges, universities, hospitals, and the state government. This diverse group of people, each representing a different skill set and a different access point in this domain, was interested in simulation not merely as a tool, but as a mechanism for building educational capacity throughout the state of Oregon. As of 2011, the OSA has facilitated the development of more than 20 simulation education programs, as well as the training of several hundred health care educators. And this great effort owes its success to the art of communication and relationships, for, as Michael notes, "we were a group of people without a history of common conversation, actually having one."

SUMMARY: FINDING A COMMON GROUND

As we continue to explore interdisciplinary education and practice to find best practices models for health care education, it is this capacity to discover, respect, and build the common ground that will support better nursing practice, and ultimately, safe and high-quality health care. Throughout the book chapters, you will learn how to develop and manage a consortium that relies on partnership and cooperation. For too long, health care education has relied on the silo model that not only separates nursing theory from nursing practice, but discourages educational and clinical agencies from sharing ideas, resources, and funds. Rather than spinning our wheels alone, repeating others' mistakes, we must look to dedicated, sophisticated business partnerships, such as consortia, to achieve quality, safe, and efficient health care.

REFERENCES

Berkow, S., Virkstis, K., Stewart, J., & Conway, L. (2009). Assessing new graduate nurse performance. *Nurse Educator, 34*(1), 17–22.

Cleland, J., Abe, K., & Rethans, J. (2009). The use of simulated patients in medical education: AMEE guide no. 411. *Medical Teacher, 31,* 477–486.

Gardner, S. F., Chamberlin, G. D., Heestand, D. E., & Stowe, C. D. (2002). Interdisciplinary didactic instruction at academic health science centers in the United States: Attitudes and barriers affecting its delivery. *Advances in Health Sciences Education, 7*(3), 179–190.

Galloway, S. J. (2009). Simulation techniques to bridge the gap between novice and competent healthcare professionals. *OJIN: The Online Journal of Issues in Nursing, 14*(2), manuscript 3.

McIntosh, C., Macario, A., Flanagan, B., & Gaba, D. M. (2006). Simulation: What does it really cost? *Simulation in Healthcare: The Journal of Society for Simulation in Healthcare, 1,* 109.

U.S. Bureau of Labor Statistics. (2010a). *Fastest growing occupations, 2008 and projected 2018.* Retrieved August 18, 2010, from http://www.bls.gov. emp/emp_table_103.htm

U.S. Bureau of Labor Statistics. (2010b). *Health care. Career guide to industries, 2010–2011 edition.* Retrieved August 18, 2010, from http://www. bls.gov/oco/cg/cgs035.htm

SUGGESTED READINGS

Beyea, S. C., Slattery, M. J., & von Reyn, L. J. (2010). Outcomes of a simulation-based nurse residency program. *Clinical Simulation in Nursing, 6*(5), e169–e175.

Block, P. (1993). *Stewardship: Choosing service over self-interest.* San Francisco, CA: Berrett-Koehler.

Gordon, E. E. (2005). *The 2010 meltdown: Solving the impending jobs crisis.* Westport, CT: Praeger.

McGaghie, W. C., Issenberg, S. B., Petrusa, E. R., & Scalese, R. J. (2010). A critical review of simulation-based medical education research: 2003–2009. *Medical Education, 44,* 50–63.

Nestel, D., Clark, S., Tabak, D., Ashwell, V., Muir, E., Paraskevas, P., & Higham, J. (2010). Defining responsibilities of simulated patients in medical education. *Society for Simulation in Health Care, 5*(3), 161–168.

Strouse, A. C. (2010). Multidisciplinary simulation centers: Promoting safe practice. *Clinical Simulation in Nursing, 6*(4), e139–e142.

TWO

Building the Consortium

Coming together is a beginning. Keeping together is progress. Working together is a success.
    —Henry Ford

*B*y design, consortia adapt to *your* needs. Structurally, they can develop as a loose affiliation of institutions, joint ventures, or formal entities with offices, staff, and multimillion dollar budgets. They can address a problem or an opportunity, spring from a grass-roots effort or serve as an offshoot of a larger grant, and extend their reach from local to global (or manage issues that are not geographically defined). Of the simulation education consortia that we interviewed, most surfaced to address nursing shortages or to increase clinical capacity or capability. Their geographical reach runs from small county initiatives to large state-wide efforts. Whatever the impetus behind your own plans for a consortium, or the focus you hope to achieve, our model aims to help you develop an adaptive, resilient partnership that can evolve according to professional or economic changes. Your first steps will include developing relationships among interested parties, formally organizing the consortium through a meeting, and laying the groundwork for a compelling narrative and shared vision.

According to Everett Rogers in *Diffusion in Innovation* (2003), innovative solutions to problems tend to run a five-stage course, from agenda-setting to routinizing (see Table 2.1).

As we progress through the steps of the simulation consortium model, you will see these stages at play. They will provide a sense of direction and assurance that events are evolving in a somewhat predictable flow.

TABLE 2.1

Five Stages of the Innovation Process

STAGE OF INNOVATION	DEFINITION
1. Setting the agenda	A problem creates a perceived need for innovation
	Example: The preparation–practice gap underprepares nursing students for professional realities
2. Matching	The problems are matched with an innovation
	Example: Clinical simulation provides a safe platform for developing and practicing bedside skills
3. Redefining or restructuring	The innovation continually becomes modified to fit the needs of a variety of organizations
	Example: A consortium forms to provide simulation opportunities to many students, rather than a few
4. Clarifying	The goals of the innovative effort become more defined and specific
	Example: Goals are set for key aspects of simulation implementation that meet the need for equipment, space, and simulation user development
5. Routinizing	The innovation becomes a part of the organizations' activity and culture. New applications are created and become operational
	Example: Simulation becomes an integral part of future innovations that push the boundaries of its original intention and benefits

Source: Roger, 2003.

DEVELOPING RELATIONSHIPS

If your consortium has branched from a large initiative, as did the Bay Area Simulation Collaborative (BASC), you likely have a group of stakeholders in place. (See Exhibits 2.1 and 2.2 for information on two consortia's different origins.)

EXHIBIT 2.1
Leveraging Established Stakeholders

BASC
KT Waxman

In 2004–2005, the California Institute for Nursing & Health Care in Oakland, CA, pulled together a group of academic and service leaders to address concerns about a predicted nursing shortage. The BASC was officially formed in 2007, with an established group of stakeholders. Today, our collaboration trains nursing faculty and nurse educators at more than 100 schools and hospitals in the San Francisco Bay Area in simulation methodology, from basic to advanced education.

EXHIBIT 2.2
Collaborating for Nursing Progress

Wright State University, Living Laboratory
Debi Sampsel

In the early 2000s, Patricia Martin, the dean of the Wright State University College of Nursing and Health, had a series of informal conversations with deans of other nursing schools about the threatening nursing shortage. In these conversations, the deans would come up with ideas to address the issue, but it seemed that again and again, the day-to-day demands of their jobs would capsize their efforts. Eventually, Dean Martin led the formation of a community collaboration to share the work and resources. They developed a small guiding group to hire an executive director and staff to examine the future of nursing in the region. This resulted in the birth of the Nursing Institute in 2004. The Living Laboratory for Simulation developed strategically from outcomes reported in the Institute's demand and supply study of the region.

If, however, you are interested in developing a consortium through a ground-up approach, you will need to build relationships. Start talking (and listening) to your colleagues, both within and outside of your institution. You can reach out through the following methods:

- Open discussions with a variety of colleagues, including hospital executives, educational institutional leaders, and community leaders, in and outside your organization
- Broach the subject with other attendees at networking events
- Use social networking platforms like Twitter and Facebook to reach a wider audience
- Post your concerns and ideas on professional bulletin boards. Even peers outside your region can have valuable information, or may be willing to brainstorm, on how to find like-minded people

These early discussions can be informal one-on-one chats. Chances are that your peers are struggling with the same issues and considering similar solutions, and they will talk about them to people they know. You will see conversations expanding to new parties and ideas coalescing around themes. And as this loose network of invested parties forms (see Figure 2.1), a core group of people will begin to identify and prioritize issues for attention, solidify their relationships, and determine their combined needs, problems, and considerations.

Figure 2.1 illustrates the typical network growth. Members of the initial core group (Arrow 1) interact with each other (Arrow 2) concerning their shared needs, problems, and considerations. Each member of this group then meets with other interested parties (Arrow 3) who, in turn, spread the word to even more interested parties. You will want to leverage that momentum to formalize your network through an organizational meeting.

Establishing the Scope of Your Consortium

Your consortium can be as small as or as vast as necessary—many of the consortia we interviewed evolved from small, localized efforts into regional or state initiatives. Those previous localized efforts in some cases had been in place for 3–5 years. The model we propose aims to develop a flexible consortium that can grow with its needs, so do not feel obliged to bite off more than you can chew. Keep the working size manageable at first.

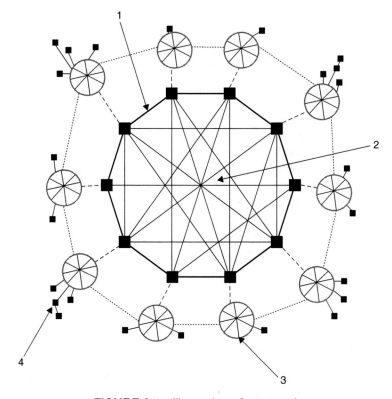

FIGURE 2.1   Illustration of a network.

Formalizing Your Partnership Through First Meetings

Your first few meetings will serve to gather and share information about simulation, discuss the focus of your group, and consider your options for moving forward. Until the partners establish an official leadership, you may wish to volunteer (or identify another) to facilitate the first few meetings. The initial meeting should include representatives from all interested institutions—these may include hospital executives, educational institution leaders, and community leaders—and aim to

- summarize the problem facing attendees;
- confirm shared interests;
- establish general goals;
- present (and request) ideas to pursue;
- declare next steps, such as fact finding and establishing consortium governance.

Encourage open communication and active listening during these early dialogues, since these activities will establish the collaborative dynamic among the stakeholders. Identify areas of agreement and examine differences of opinion. Use your time to perform the following activities:

- Define the initiative's boundaries, such as geographical, scope of work, or groups being affected or involved
- Share general information about simulation, including evidence-based data, to be certain that all participants are on the same page
- Address the initiative's benefits for participants
- Consider funding. These monies may not be identified yet, but the required resources can be estimated so that members can get a sense of the financial needs
- Identify tools and measurements for evaluating results and outcomes
- Propose a governance structure that outlines roles and responsibilities

You will also need to assign someone to coordinate a needs assessment that will gather information about the current state of simulation education in your region. This needs assessment will establish the consortium's baseline for its discussion of broad goals. End the first meeting by identifying next steps and assigning responsibilities—these may include gathering data for a needs assessment; brainstorming ideas for an initial project plan, vision, and mission; and establishing a governance structure. See Exhibit 2.3 for a sample agenda.

Gathering Data

Members of any group project can get caught up in the excitement of developing an innovative solution—and this energy is a good thing. It is the fuel that drives the engine of growth and commitment. According to Rogers (2003), however, we often spend too little time considering the consequences of our proposed changes. Rogers advises consortia to thoroughly research other efforts to develop simulation centers, learning from both their successes and their failures.

EXHIBIT 2.3
Sample Agenda for the First Meeting

    I. Overall goals of the simulation center initiative
   II. Similarities or areas of overlap between the simulation
       center proposal and other health care or educational
       initiatives in your region
  III. Health care–related demographics of the region
  IV. Benefits of participation to consortium members
   V. Funding sources, or request for funding needed
  VI. Summary of initial research on simulation

       A. Advantages of simulation
       B. Challenges
       C. Lessons others have learned

  VII. Methods of evaluation and outcomes
 VIII. Discussion
  IX. Next steps

As soon as possible, establish a coordinator or a committee to gather information about simulation, including the following:

- Literature review
- Types of simulation equipment and application
- Benefits and challenges of simulation education
- Outcomes and measures
- Funding

This process may take 2–3 months to complete, but the coordinator or committee will analyze and share the findings with the consortium through a report or presentation. Task your committee with collecting information from such typical sources as books, research articles, published surveys, and the Internet, but also

- survey members of your consortium on the status of their simulation education capabilities;
- interview experienced simulation users and experts;
- visit active simulation centers to get a first-hand perspective of the process and experience;
- perform demand–supply studies of nurses needed in the region;

- collect cost information on starting up a simulation center;
- identify the benefits of using simulation methodology.

The consortium will use this information—which may take 2–3 months to collect—to organize its participants' energy into goals and plans for implementation.

The committee should develop an approach to information gathering that is both structured and open to exploring unknown leads and variations. This approach may seem contradictory, but it attacks the issue logically *and* intuitively. It uncovers the breadth of data available while allowing for a deeper, more complex understanding of the issue. Questions to guide your initial research include the following:

- Who else has accomplished or is working toward goals similar to ours? When did they begin their simulation project?
- What were their successes and challenges?
- Were their needs, resources, and partnerships similar to ours? Were their outcomes similar to the ones we hope to achieve? If they differ, how and why so? What can we learn from the differences and similarities?
- Which of their lessons apply to our situation?
- Can we contact them for an interview or visit?

You may discover a series of repeated findings or variances during this phase of research, but this information is important. Repetition will provide confidence in your conclusions, whereas variances provide new information worth exploring.

In addition to such specific tasks as meetings and research, consortia build community through high-level work, such as developing compelling stories and shared vision.

THE COMPELLING STORY

All of the task-oriented work your consortium members do contribute to your group's "compelling story." In this context, a compelling story articulates the focus of the group, as well as the benefits and challenges of its mission. It begins through an iterative progress, with a conversation about common needs, concerns, and solutions. As research continues and relationships grow, discussions become richer because you are communicating at two levels—the abstract and the concrete. Data will contextualize abstract concepts, such as "nursing shortage," and inspire creative thinking with real solutions.

Your members will hone the consortium's scope by discussing its parameters, asking questions, and providing feedback, and the story becomes more meaningful and easier to articulate clearly. As one consortium coordinator put it, "The story became more compelling to me first and then to others as we kept talking. For example, I was able to answer more questions clearly and state what I thought the benefits would be for our region and how we could consider going about implementation. As a result, others were able to do the same and, over time, we developed this ongoing 'compelling story.'"

SHARED VISION

In the context of a consortium, "shared vision" does not mean "complete agreement"; rather, it provides one, collective response in service to the individual needs of all consortium partners. It respects their different goals, while offering a common aspiration to rally around. Each partner can interpret this shared vision differently. For instance, Table 2.2 shows the different needs met by partners' common belief that simulation education advances the nursing profession.

Recognizing these small but important differences will become important, as the consortium becomes formalized, and develops and implements a strategic plan. By being aware of each partner's specific needs, the consortium can respond appropriately and supportively. This process helps the consortium grow stronger and invest in the needs of the community.

TABLE 2.2
Needs Met by the Shared Vision

PARTNER TYPE	OPPORTUNITIES PROVIDED BY CONSORTIUM
Postsecondary University	Interdisciplinary research opportunities among academic and clinical partners in a regional area
Critical access hospital	Staff access to expensive, invaluable simulation technology
Career technical center	Early experience working with mannequins and scenarios for high-school students

(continued)

TABLE 2.2
Needs Met by the Shared Vision (*continued*)

PARTNER TYPE	OPPORTUNITIES PROVIDED BY CONSORTIUM
Acute care hospital	Integration of simulation laboratory with other innovative health care practices that lead to process improvement in programs and delivery of services
Community college	Use of simulation technology to reinforce curricula and attainment of higher NCLEX scores
Area health education center	Engaging clinical rotations and access to technology for interns in a rural region

LESSONS LEARNED

■ Understanding the needs of each partner in a consortium is a continuous process. They change as the context of their environment changes.

■ No one person or organization has the *right* vision. It takes input from all to develop common ground, understanding, and commitment.

■ A shared vision does not mean everyone has *exactly* the same interpretation; it only means that they find something in it that attracts them and meets their needs. Take the time to understand each person's interpretation.

■ Periodically track each partner's commitment level. Engagement of all partners is critical to success.

■ Trust builds over time and through respectful collaboration. Working together allows partners to see each other in a variety of settings and situations.

■ Despite our best efforts, we may experience unintended consequences of our actions—both positive and negative. For ideas on preparing for and addressing these consequences, turn to Chapter 8.

SUMMARY

These early steps—networking, gathering participants and data, and creating a compelling story and a shared vision—may seem simple or intuitive, but attending to them thoughtfully will provide the consortium's work with its foundation. These steps establish the sense of community, respect, and collaboration that fuels the consortium through its planning, implementing, re-visioning and adapting, and sustaining stages.

REFERENCES

consortium. (n.d.). *Merriam-Webster's dictionary of law.* Retrieved August 29, 2010, from http://dictionary.reference.com/browse/consortium

Rogers, E. M. (2003). *Diffusion of innovations* (5th ed.). New York, NY: Free Press.

SUGGESTED READINGS

Barabasi, A.-L. (2002). *Linked: The new science of networks.* Cambridge, MA: Perseus.

Shirky, C. (2008). *Here comes everybody: The power of organizing without organizations.* New York, NY: Penguin.

Senge, P., Smith, B., Kruschwitz, N., Laura, J., & Schley, S. (2008). *Necessary revolution: How individuals and organizations are working together to create a sustainable world.* New York, NY: Doubleday.

Weisbord, M. R. (1992). *Discovering common ground: How future search conferences bring people together to achieve breakthrough innovation, empowerment, shared vision, and collaborative action.* San Francisco, CA: Berrett-Kohler.

THREE

Leading and Managing the Consortium

Good leaders must first become servants.
—Robert Greenleaf

Now that the consortium has come together, you will need to provide its members with definition and structure for working together. In this chapter, we will examine the roles and responsibilities of the steering committee, other committees, the project coordinator, and the simulation consultant—the consortium's formal leadership structure. In addition, we will describe the informal leadership and contribution that each member potentially brings with them. Together, these two facets of leadership charge the energy needed to set goals, provide direction, take action, and implement the simulation consortium model.

STEWARDSHIP: LEADERSHIP THROUGH SERVICE

In their bestselling book, *The Leadership Challenge*, James Kouzes and Barry Posner (2007) suggest, "to get a feel for the true essence of leadership, assume that everyone who works with you is a volunteer." These words are especially true throughout the world of consortium leadership, since most members choose to invest their organizations, as well as their own time and energies, in the work of the consortium. This volunteerism defines the most effective leadership style for this type of partnership: servant leadership, or stewardship.

Peter Block (2003) defines stewardship as the willingness to be accountable for the well-being of the larger organization by operating in service rather than in control. He notes that an organization experiences authentic service when four conditions are met:

1. A balance of power exists
2. The larger community serves as the primary commitment
3. Each person joins in defining the purpose and culture of the organization
4. A balanced and equitable distribution of rewards exists

Creating a governing structure that encourages all members to contribute will help ensure that your consortium lives these conditions. The structure may depend on your consortium's origins: If your consortium branched off from a larger initiative, you may have other entities to answer to. For instance, the consortium managing the Simulation Center at Fairbanks Hall, which is a collaboration between Indiana University Health (which owns or is affiliated with more than 20 hospitals and health centers in Indiana) and Indiana University's Schools of Medicine and Nursing, has an overriding executive committee that includes members from all participating organizations (Exhibit 3.1).

EXHIBIT 3.1

A Flexible, Top–Down Approach

The Simulation Center at Fairbanks Hall
Scott A. Engum, MD

Our overarching executive and governance committee comprised representatives from each of our three partners—Indiana University Health, Indiana University School of Medicine, and Indiana University School of Nursing. They determined the global mission, vision, goals, and funding allocations for this collaborative effort to ensure the center was state of the art and timely in its completion.

This committee established an interdisciplinary operating committee that included a project management company, health care system administrative leaders, educators from the three entities, and business management personnel who oversaw all planning, ordering, and construction-related activities. As the project neared completion, liaisons were established for each entity and these individuals drive the educational simulation goals of their respective organizations, while enhancing collaborative opportunities among partners. The liaisons are members of our leadership group, which meets every other week to review center-related issues and drive strategic planning. We also have regular management meetings, which include the center coordinator, technicians, and administrative support personnel, to regularly review event schedules and complete the feedback loop on previous simulation events.

For most of our consortium contributors, however, large, state-wide initiatives grew out of local/regional initiatives. It seems like state-wide initiatives have not yet been organized well enough to demonstrate success stories.

ESTABLISHING YOUR ORGANIZATIONAL STRUCTURE

Depending on the size and scope of your consortium, your members may choose a formal leadership structure with many layers and defined roles and responsibilities—state-wide efforts, in particular, tend to be more formally organized, with connections to state board of nursing guidelines. Many consortia prefer a less circumscribed organization. Of the consortium leaders we interviewed, we found similar elements among their governing structures:

- A board or executive committee that makes and implements major organizational decisions
- An expert in simulation, to provide guidance on technologies, equipment, and applications
- A steering/operating committee or advisory group, comprising of high-level stakeholders who provide guidance on objectives, strategy, budget and resource allocation, and other major decisions
- Support staff, including a project director or similar position, to coordinate organizational design responsibilities and implement decisions taken by the steering committee

The consortia also developed committees (or established relationships with existing committees) for specific goals or projects, either ongoing or ad hoc. In developing the consortium's structure, keep your stewardship role in mind—maintain the balance of power, encourage each member's contributions, and serve the community fairly.

Governing Board or Executive Committee

501(c)(3) organizations require a formal structure that usually involves a governing board, as spelled out in their bylaws. (For examples of consortiums with formal and informal structures, see Exhibits 3.2 and 3.3.) This entity often goes by many names, including "board of directors," "executive board," and "executive team." Essentially, this group consists of key stakeholders who jointly oversee the activities of the consortium. It typically makes decisions concerning high-level matters outside the operation of the consortium,

---

EXHIBIT 3.2
A Formal, 501(c)3 Structure

Oregon Simulation Alliance
Michael Seropian, MD, and Bonnie Driggers

We were the first simulation consortium to seek and achieve 501(c)3 status. Similar groups had developed relationships with hospitals and schools, community colleges, and universities, but few had the breadth and depth of the OSA across communities and statewide, and as such, we felt that our organization needed a formal structure. It turns out that, because we focused on developing a broad, strong foundation with a multiprofessional board and flexible infrastructure, simulation education in Oregon has had a wider spread and greater depth than other consortiums in terms of implementation and capacity. Subscriptions and grants fund the operations of the OSA, not an individual entity. An opt-out program, eligibility for subscription to the OSA, automatically includes all health care organizations and collaboratives in the state, such as the OCNE, among its subscribers to create a network of collaborative associations that feed into this large, dynamic alliance.

EXHIBIT 3.3
An Informal Structure

Southeastern Indiana
Dave Galle

In Southeast Indiana, ours is an informal structure. We have a steering committee (made up of representatives from each of the participating organizations) and a simulation advisory group backed by a support staff team. The Community Education Coalition, a partnership of education, business, and community leaders that I direct, received a EcO15 (*Economic Opportunities through Education by 2015*) grant. We, in turn, provided funding to other organizations, but we have not created a formal organizational structure.

such as creating mission, vision, and value statements; setting goals; allocating resources; and approving budgets.

Steering Committee

The steering or operating committee, or advisory group, provides their expertise on achieving the goals of the consortium. It includes representatives from each of the major stakeholders who provide guidance on objectives, strategy, budget and resource allocation, and other major decisions. Major stakeholders could include county, regional, or state-wide organizations; related health care organizations; and potential funders, depending upon the goals and scope of the consortium. In some instances, public sector leaders, research organizations, workforce investment boards, employers, advocacy groups, and service providers have joined together to form steering committees. Such committees can include funders who collaborate in a variety of ways, based on agreed-upon principles, priorities, and strategies. Responsibilities of the steering committee might include the following:

- Providing input into the vision, mission, and values of the consortium
- Reviewing the strategic plan and offering recommendations for changes, if necessary

- Advocating for simulation education and supporting the consortium's initiatives
- Monitoring and reviewing project statuses
- Providing assistance to projects as requested
- Managing project scope to ensure that the needs of stakeholders are being met
- Making budget recommendations

Content Expert(s)

This person or committee provides input on the current state of simulation education. He or she advises on equipment, capabilities, and simulation pedagogies, especially during the consortium's early days. As the consortium grows and develops its own content experts, this person may assume a more advisory capacity. Responsibilities of the content expert might include the following:

- Providing data and input on clinical simulation needs
- Providing input to the strategic plan
- Implementing the plan as it impacts their organization
- Reporting progress in task force meetings
- Sharing promising practices with other consortium members
- Encouraging new innovations and practices that may fit with the mission and vision of the consortium

Support Staff Team

The support staff team shoulders organizational design responsibilities and leads the steering committee through development of the strategic plan, the professional development plan, and the strategic plan audit. A support staff team might include the project director and an administrative coordinator to arrange meetings and webinars and to perform any other administrative functions of the consortium. Depending upon the scope of the effort (regional, state, or national), the size of the support team will vary. The support team's responsibilities might include the following:

- Facilitating steering committee and task force meetings
- Providing technical assistance and direction

■ Ensuring regular communication between the executive committee, steering committee, and consortium participants
■ Designing and implementing key elements of the strategic plan, including the following:
  • Infrastructure
  • Programs
  • Professional development plan
  • Strategy plan evaluation

Your consortium will find a structure that meets its specific needs. And as your number of partnerships grows, and your consortium activities expand their complexity, you will need to form committees for specific activities, such as funding and sustainability, programming, or simulation research.

DEFINE YOUR VISION, MISSION, AND VALUES

Once your leadership and organization is in place, your consortium can expand its shared vision into formal vision, mission, and core values statements. These statements, developed through deliberation and collaborative discussion, assist a consortium in maintaining focus on stewardship and course toward its goals, particularly when it needs to make difficult decisions, dissolve an impasse, manage "project creep," or resolve confusion among its members. Steven Haines (1995) shares the following definitions of these statements:

■ *Vision:* Articulates your members' shared hopes, dreams, and image of the consortium's future
■ *Mission:* Identifies the rationale behind your consortium, its goals, and its audience
■ *Core Values:* Guide the consortium's regular activities and create its organizational culture

Your steering committee can collaborate to develop early drafts of these statements. One helpful exercise asks each member to write down their own versions to share with the group. The facilitator or the steering committee chair can use these draft statements to lead the group into a discussion that builds ideas for consensus. Or, your consortium may prefer to charge a small team to draw up drafts to present to the group for review and approval. It is critical, however, that you encourage input from your participants. Such statements can seem abstract, particularly when contrasted with the down-and-dirty work of the consortium, so wrangling with the concepts will invest individuals more strongly in these ideals than if they were simply declared by the leadership.

Mission Statement

By defining our customers, our products and services, and our unique purpose, a mission statement can motivate and provide clarity to other key stakeholders and the community at large. Facilitate the discussion of your mission statement by asking the four questions that, according to Peter Block (1993), a mission statement answers:

1. Who is our audience?
2. What products and/or services do we provide them?
3. What is the unique value that we add?
4. What will be the results of our work together?

To develop ownership and commitment among your consortium members, ask each participant to answer these questions individually before discussing them with the group. This group dialogue will foment a richer, more advanced understanding of the ideals and goals the consortium seeks to enact. Once you have drafted a near-final mission statement, review it with members of your audience to be certain that it meets their needs.

Vision Statement

A vision statement articulates a high-level statement of where your consortium wants to go. By capturing your partnership's ideal future, your vision statement focuses all of your organizational planning. If your mission statement sets your consortium's core compass, your vision statement provides the direction for the work of your consortium. Ask yourself questions like the following:

■ Where do you see the consortium in 3 years, and again in 5 years?
■ What does the consortium want to be known for?

Answers will help you define your consortium's direction, which will, in turn, impact your decisions and resource allocation.

Core Values

In *Act Made Simple,* Russ Harris (2009) states that core values guide and support an organization's conduct on an ongoing basis. They articulate the behaviors we wish to exhibit in our work to achieve the vision and mission, and reflect the consortium's stewardship role. Establishing core values within the consortium is a shared dialogue; all members should contribute. Ask broad questions such as the following:

- What do we value?
- What values should our consortium represent and what attributes should be visible to both our internal and external community?

Table 3.1 depicts a sampling of core values and the rationale behind adopting them.

TABLE 3.1
Rationale Behind Specific Core Values

CORE VALUE	RATIONALE
Cooperation	The simulation center project requires us to work together. With our limited resources, we cannot accomplish our goals by working separately. Cooperation will also allow us to draw upon the creative ideas and diversity of thinking within our group
High involvement	Consortium partners must be highly involved with the business of the group, especially when it comes to major decisions. You do not want to find out too late that an expensive decision does not meet the needs of other stakeholders
Learning	As an organization dedicated to simulation education, we value learning because we know that we must continuously improve, particularly in the area of patient care and safety

(continued)

TABLE 3.1
Rationale Behind Specific Core Values (*continued*)

CORE VALUE	RATIONALE
Gratitude	We are thankful for the opportunity to build the simulation center that funding has given us. We demonstrate our gratitude by creating excellence in all that we do
Making a difference	As a result of the simulation technology in our educational programs, we will be able to practice both common and unusual procedures that will make a significant difference to our students, health care professionals, and patients. Our students and health care professionals will be more confident and competent
Service	Serving our audience and meeting their needs is paramount to our mission. The benefits of simulation education align well with improving patient care and safety

How do the consortium's regular activities reflect these values? Let us take a look:

Cooperation. Rather than asking each partner to develop scenarios independently, the consortium has decided to develop a regional library of simulation scenarios that would benefit all stakeholders. They will meet to discuss scenarios needed and assign responsibility to those who have the expertise to complete them.

High involvement. The consortium has begun to look at sustaining the benefits of their simulation education project. The steering committee will examine the benefits and identify activities that they want to maintain. They will determine and allocate resources to maintain those activities, while developing other funding sources and strategies. Although they have not yet completed their work, the consortium displays a high degree of engagement and commitment to concluding the process with viable recommendations.

Learning. The consortium has established a professional development plan for simulation users within their audience. The plan is comprehensive and based on needs identified by the consultant and users. It includes a combination of learning activities that facilitate continuous learning of simulation education methods: books, workshops, webinars, online training modules, and technical assistance with equipment suppliers. Through national research projects and exposure, the consortium has encouraged clinical simulation leaders to participate in educational opportunities.

Gratitude. The consortium provides feedback to funders of the simulation education complex on project outcomes and benefits. It e-mails newsletters to key stakeholders and the broader network to keep them apprised of current activity and progress towards goals. Another option includes acknowledging the funding and support of the project in any presentations or publications.

Making a difference. Monthly reports can include success stories on how the use of simulation technology has improved the confidence level of students and health care professionals. In addition, the narratives of promising practices are routinely shared and available for all simulation users to retrieve and use as appropriate for their needs.

Service. Research shows that simulation education increases confidence and competence of its users. It provides them opportunity to practice procedures that increase their knowledge and skill levels to provide better patient care.

Clearly, consortium activities can affirm its stated values in both small and large ways. As these values are demonstrated in day-to-day practice, they begin to shape the culture that surrounds them.

Vision, mission, and values provide direction and clarity; they work like magnets to pull the consortium back to task, while allowing us to adapt and grow our orbit as appropriate.

USING MISSION, VISION, AND CORE VALUES

The vision and mission statements can help a consortium manage project creep—a natural by-product of any initiative. Some project creep can actually enrich the direction of the consortium, but other project creep can derail consortium efforts from their goals. As resources are pulled in various directions, check whether each effort supports the vision and mission statements. At least once a year, the steering committee should review the vision and mission statements to ensure that they still meet the needs of its audience. Sometimes changing just a few words can articulate different and powerful messages to the consortium about its position and direction.

How does a consortium lead its members to invest in its mission, vision, and core values?

1. Ask each member to develop and share their own versions of vision, mission, and value for the consortium. This dialogue respects each member's input, encourages communication, and enriches the final statements.
2. Ask each member to discuss their organization's audience and the product or service they provide to that audience. This dialogue, performed collectively, can reveal the abilities, interests, and uniqueness available to the consortium, thereby building an inventory of strengths that the consortium can call upon as needed.
3. Values drive behavior, so when difficult decisions arise, ask your leaders and members to consider which priorities drive the consortium's activities.
4. Occasionally take time to reflect on the direction and activities of the consortium. Are they serving the larger community in the way that you want?
5. Ask the question, "Are stakeholders and partners receiving the benefits that we identified?" Is there a fair distribution of rewards?

This type of active dialogue—one that encourages input as well as healthy disagreement—engages participants in the work of the statements and ensures that they continue to meet the needs of the consortium's partners and its community, even if that population changes over time.

Managing Growth

Your mission and vision statements can also help you manage growth. Despite the temptation to quickly increase the size of your consortium, an unwieldy organization cannot accomplish good work efficiently. If your governing and administrative structure does not adapt at an equal rate, your efforts will suffer. But your governing statements, along with the strategic plan and goals, can provide boundaries and considerations for expansion. The steering committee can use them to identify secondary or tertiary organizations or initiatives that might be impacted by your work and/or able to provide assets to grow the effort. They can also disqualify the organizations that would not fall under the reach of your work, advance your goals, or live your core values.

Managing Project Creep

Project creep—that slow, often unnoticeable expansion of scope—can sneak up on you quietly, so established governing statements can also help you assess and manage it. Project creep reflects the synergy effect of an expanded network; occasionally, any system will generate unpredictable advantages or disadvantages. Some kinds of project creep can benefit your consortium's work by increasing the rewards of your output. Other project creep drains resources and attention. First, assess new opportunities for their fit with the guidelines set by your statements; if appropriate, evaluate the return on investment (ROI) against your consortium's capacity to take on this additional work. If the ROI is significant, your consortium may consider pursuing the opportunity as a wise investment.

LESSONS LEARNED

- Vision, mission, and values do not develop in one sitting. They emerge over time, from dialogue among consortium members.
- The personal vision, mission, and values of each consortium member ensure greater engagement of the entire consortium. As each consortium member shares their thoughts, they will invariably impact the other members' views: This process leads to a deeper and richer understanding of these governing statements by the whole group.
- Periodically evaluate the engagement level of the consortium and take actions to keep them involved.

SUMMARY

Developing mission, vision, and core values statements that foster a service-oriented leadership enables your consortium to define its scope and direction, encourages ownership among its members, and supports its educational community. In the next chapter, we will examine ways that collaboration helps a consortium continue this work.

REFERENCES

Block, P. (1993, 2003). *Stewardship: Choosing service over self-interest.* San Francisco, CA: Berrett-Koehler.

Haines, S. G. (1995). *Successful strategic planning.* Menlo Park, CA: Course Technology Crisp.

Harris, R. (2009). *ACT made simple: An easy-to-read primer on acceptance and commitment therapy.* Oakland, CA: New Harbinger.

Kouzes, J., & Posner, B. (2007). *The leadership challenge* (4th ed.). San Francisco, CA: Jossey-Bass.

SUGGESTED READINGS

Buckingham, M., & Clifton, D. O. (2001). *Now, discover your strengths.* New York, NY: Free Press.

Covey, S. M. R. (2006). *The speed of trust.* New York, NY: Free Press.

Kotter, J. P. (1996). *Leading change.* Boston, MA: Harvard Business School Press.

Rath, T., & Conchi, B. (2008). *Strengths-based leadership: Great leaders, teams, and why people follow.* New York, NY: Gallup.

Studer, Q. (2003). *Hardwiring Excellence: Purpose-worthwhile work making a difference.* Baltimore, MD: Fire Starter.

FOUR

Collaborating With Others

If you have an apple and I have an apple and we exchange these apples, then you and I still have one apple. But if you have an idea and I have an idea and we exchange these ideas, then each of us will have two ideas.
—George Bernard Shaw

Collaboration threads throughout the entire process of the simulation consortium model: from the first sharing of ideas and concerns during the building phase, through the development of high-level governing concepts and plans, to reaching the goal of sustainability. At every point along the way, the model turns on the axis of collaboration. It is so important that we have dedicated an entire chapter to the process, hoping that if consortium leaders understand how collaboration builds shared respect and ownership, as well as how to facilitate it, you can ensure that consortium activities and messages support the goals of the entire community.

WHY COLLABORATE?

As Strauss (2002) describes it succinctly, collaboration happens when "you need to get the support and agreement of others before you take action of some kind" (p. 2). Collaboration not only builds a sense of community and ownership, but it also offers a richer set of ideas and resources than that found in individual efforts. Successful collaboration depends on communication, leverages the deep resources of complex, interdependent relationships, and results in improved outcomes.

Communication Connects

Across the board, our consortium leaders emphasized good communication strategies. Your partners can only experience candid dialogue if each one has all of the information available. As your consortium grows in number and complexity, it becomes difficult to maintain clear lines of communication, to listen carefully, and to manage disagreements. But patience and flexibility can help. So can technology! Most of the consortia we interviewed apprised partners through newsletters and dedicated Web sites or pages, but they also provided opportunities for groups to speak, listen, and share ideas in real time. Internet and telephone conferences alleviate some scheduling challenges, but if possible, many people prefer face-to-face meetings that provide deeper engagement and build richer, more "real" interpersonal bonds. (Exhibit 4.1 details the Southeast Indiana Health Care Consortium's efforts to communicate effectively.) Your major stakeholders can include a representative in each of the major committees, to serve as a liaison, ensure transparency, and identify opportunities to share knowledge.

EXHIBIT 4.1
Effective Communication

Southeastern Indiana Health Care Consortium
Dave Galle

We make a point of contacting people outside of regular meetings, asking for their new ideas and concerns. We manage the relationships on a day-to-day basis and make sure that those lines of communication are open. We pay attention to where we think each of the partners is at in their goals, and we let them know proactively. It is important to listen to people's needs and respond quickly and appropriately.

Effective collaboration also requires specific communication regarding the scope of the project and the investment of your partners' time and resources. When assigning a task or project, include the following information:

- Expected time frame
- Expected hours to complete the task
- Project goals
- Deadlines
- Expected input or support from other partners (make sure that these partners are aware of the expectations)
- Specific deliverables

See Exhibit 4.2 for an example of a request to the steering committee to collaborate in the development of a strategic plan.

EXHIBIT 4.2
Request for Collaboration

Sample Person A and Sample Person B will be organizing a task force, consisting of members of the consortium organizations, to begin development of a strategic plan. We ask your support in identifying one or two members of your organization to participate in the strategic planning process. We estimate that the project will require three or four meetings (10–12 hours in total) over a 2- to 3-month period. The task force will return to the steering committee in three months with a draft of a strategic plan that will include the following:

- A scan of the regional health care environment
- A description of current simulation use in our region
- A description of our expectations for simulation use in our region
- The strategies to move us toward our goal
- A project timetable and resource requirements to implement the strategies
- The benefits we expect upon using simulation education pedagogy

We will send a copy of the draft to you prior to our next meeting for your review.

This request outlines the responsibilities of the organizers of the strategic planning process, the expectations of the consortium leaders, and the time frame for completion.

Streamline your communications as best as you can, but be prepared for misunderstandings to happen and to learn from them. If appropriate, you can even turn the situation into a collaborative exercise by discussing the causes and effects with your partners, and how to ensure that the problem does not happen again. Over time, you will adopt a balance and appreciation of mistakes as "gifts" that teach lessons and encourage adaptability.

Diversity Rewards

By their nature and design, consortia can develop a web of highly interdependent relationships. Each partner has a separate relationship with each of the other partners, forming a vast interdependent connectivity, with each member bringing different agendas, needs, resources, and goals. These partners can differ in many tangible respects, such as location or type of organization (i.e., critical access hospital, acute care hospital, secondary and postsecondary educational institutions, or nonprofit organizations). This complex network means that the success or failure of one partner depends upon the others. Collaboration allows consortium leaders to balance the differences among the participating organizations to set common goals, solve common problems, and ensure overall success. If managed appropriately, the diversity among the partners allows the group to share resources and expertise in different areas, while accommodating individual deficiencies. Leaders can facilitate that inclusive discussion by maintaining an open dialogue, encouraging diverse opinions, and managing disagreements constructively. Exhibit 4.3 illustrates the Oregon Consortium for Nursing Education's successful conflict-management style.

EXHIBIT 4.3
Managing Conflict Constructively

The Oregon Consortium for Nursing Education
Paula Gubrud-Howe

For many years, the state of Oregon had a very fractured health care community. Most of the health care data and funding were focused on the urban centers, to the exclusion of our large rural population. An almost 20-year rift also existed between our state's schools of nursing and community college nursing programs over the issue of entry into practice, so neither group was talking to the other. But in 2001, when rumblings about the national nursing shortage began to appear, Dr. Chris Tanner performed a state-wide, comprehensive study that forecasted a 50% vacancy rate by 2020.

With the urgency of the situation so clearly defined, these warring factions were forced to quit fighting and develop consensus on how best to prepare for the shortage and rehabilitate the nursing profession. We needed to create a whole new culture of collaboration.

We have been very intentional in learning how to engage in constructive conflict. The OCNE developed guiding principles to help define our behaviors with each other. Regular communication is integral to helping members feel invested: We have annual meetings, as well as monthly telephone conferences, and a yearly leadership retreat. We publish a newsletter and share information on the Web site. We have small conflicts all the time, but we have learned to consider them as challenges. We remind ourselves of our long-term goals and focus on solving problems, rather than blaming others.

Outcomes Improve

By implementing communication systems and strategies that encourage discussion and manage conflict, while drawing upon the diverse perspectives and resources of your partners, consortium leaders can ensure improved outcomes. This collaboration allows members to reduce the workload investment, but share the profits. Table 4.1 shows the outcome of the Southeastern Indiana Regional Health Care Consortium's collaborative work.

By facilitating the input of each partner, the consortium leaders fostered a sense of inclusion and ownership in the work, while accommodating the diversity of opinions.

TABLE 4.1
Differences Among Plans

PLAN ITEM	ORIGINAL PROPOSAL	FINAL PLAN	BENEFITS
Number of locations	Four simulation laboratories and two mobile units	Ten simulation laboratories, with control rooms and debriefing rooms; no mobile units	Increased involvement of all partners; reduced scheduling problems

(continued)

TABLE 4.1

Differences Among Plans (*continued*)

PLAN ITEM	ORIGINAL PROPOSAL	FINAL PLAN	BENEFITS
Staff support	One technician	Technical capability at each site integrated into current staff	Integrated simulation technology in current local work versus reliance on a regional staff
Balance of power	Central location and two satellite locations would have most of the resources	Each of 14 locations was involved in the process of planning and making decisions. Based on the needs of each location, ownership of simulation equipment and assets varied	Increased ownership, commitment, and rewards
Commitment to the larger community	Broad-based and dependent upon the execution of plan	Development of regional simulation scenario library; memorandum of understanding with each location on use of equipment and assets; broad professional development plan covering all locations and close to 100 faculty/ professionals; goals set for each location to deliver simulation training and education	Increased capability across the region
Decision making	Centralized	Decentralized, yet focus on regional needs as appropriate	Blended decisions serve both regional and local needs
Cost	On budget	Below budget	More cost-effective overall

PLAN FOR COLLABORATION

The idea of collaboration seems simple; the implementation is not always so. The temptation to make a unilateral decision or push an agenda can be nearly irresistible, particularly when schedules are pressing. Your best defense? Examine your consortium-building process early on. (See Exhibit 4.4 for the OSA's strategies for building collaborative relationships into a consortium's business plan.) Fit collaborative opportunities into every step, and stick with your plan. Remember that it is not a consortium if the activities bear the input of and benefit only a few partners. For ideas for collaborative opportunities throughout the process, see the Appendix at the end of this chapter.

EXHIBIT 4.4
Building Collaboration into the Business Plan

The Oregon Simulation Alliance
Michael Seropian, MD, and Bonnie Driggers

Early on, one of the OSA's RFP processes ensured that each applicant built collaboration into its business plan. The process required applicants to belong to some form of collaborative entity, and to outline specifically how that collaboration operates. But funding does not a collaborative make. It is not a replacement for a working relationship, nor is it, in itself, a value. It is how you work together to use that money, and how you set yourself up for success, that defines the value of your consortium. We saw a lot of "paper collaborations;" entities that united solely for the purpose of a grant, and had little experience of how to work together at the ground level. When the grant was over, there was a risk that the local relationships would end. That fortunately did not happen, as many of the collaboratives still flourish today.

The OSA's planning process ensured that each collaborative effort focused on a mission or goal: framing it this way forced applicants to develop a realistic collaborative process to achieve that goal. We recommend that collaboratives define themselves early. Frey's Levels of Collaboration Scale

(2006) is a good resource to help parties define what *kind* of collaboration they expect and wish to aim for. It could be as simple as a "network" sharing information or as complex as an elaborate collaboration sharing funding and decision making. We have found that defining the type of collaboration makes the crafting of a mission and vision much easier.

How do you know when a decision or task requires collaboration? Strauss developed a helpful decision-making model that advises leaders to consider two aspects of collaboration—the level of ownership and the level of involvement required—as follows:

1. When stakeholder buy-in is important, the expertise lies within the group, and you have available time to work together, building consensus through collaboration is your best option.
2. When stakeholder buy-in is not very important, the expertise is readily available, and time is critical, making decisions with less collaboration may be more appropriate. For example, stakeholders may not hold certain issues in high priority, so the impact of making an independent decision would be minimal. Work closely with stakeholders to understand the types of decisions and issues that are important to them. Occasionally, the expertise lies in a single, easily identified individual, either inside or outside the group. In these situations, leaders can make decisions and take action without the group's consent, perhaps including information that substantiates the individual's expertise in your communications.

LESSONS LEARNED

- Working in a collaborative manner requires seeking common ground in our decisions and actions. Rather than considering simply our own needs, our focus shifts towards the broad community or consortium.
- As the consortium grows and works together over time, the unique strengths and assets of the group become clearer and more accessible to others.
- Because a collaborative effort like a consortium requires greater interdependency, the consortium may make some mistakes

more easily. Openly acknowledging your occasional mistakes builds trust.

■ Collaboration is not a panacea; it simply provides both greater benefits and challenges for those who choose to work in this manner. Over the long term, it can also ensure better quality of relationships and outcomes.

SUMMARY

Collaboration works best as a *process*, not as an end goal. It allows better working relationships and better outcomes, and ensures that your work meets the needs of the entire community. Use the simulation consortium model to build and encourage opportunities for collaboration, as detailed in the Appendix to this chapter.

REFERENCE

Strauss, D., & Layton T. C. (2002). *How to make collaboration work: Powerful ways to build consensus, solve problems, and make decisions.* San Francisco, CA: Berett-Kohler.

SUGGESTED READINGS

Frey, B. B., Lohmeier, J. H., Lee, S. W., & Tollefson, N. (2006). Measuring collaboration among grant partners. *American Journal of Evaluation, 27,* 383–392.

Gray, B. (1989). *Collaborating: Finding common ground for multiparty problems.* San Franscisco, CA: Jossey-Bass.

Mattlessich, P. W., Murray-Close, M., & Monsey, B. R. (2001). *Collaboration: What makes it work* (2nd ed.). Saint Paul, MN: Amherst H. Wilder Foundation.

Pfeffer, J., & Sutton, R. I. (2000). *The knowing-doing gap: How smart companies turn knowledge into action.* Boston, MA: Harvard Business School Press.

Surowiecki, J. (2004). *The wisdom of crowds: Why the many are smarter than the few and how collective wisdom shapes business, economies, societies, and nations.* New York, NY: Doubleday.

The Peter Drucker Foundation for Nonprofit Management. (2002). *Meeting the collaboration challenge workbook: Developing strategic alliances between nonprofit organizations and businesses.* San Francisco, CA: Jossey-Bass.

Appendix: Collaborative Opportunities Throughout the Simulation Consortium Model

The following lists detail the many opportunities for collaboration in each step of the simulation consortium model. Use these lists to build collaboration into your activities and processes from the beginning.

BUILDING THE CONSORTIUM

- Discuss the magnitude of the opportunity or threat behind the consortium.
- Seek out those with a common interest in the opportunity.
- Organize a meeting to discuss common needs.
- Document meetings and forward minutes, including action items, to key stakeholders.
- Explore differences of opinion.
- Collect additional information to clarify issues.
- Provide forums for further dialogue and feedback on ideas.
- Develop and present a proposal for discussion.
- Develop and share personal visions.

LEADING AND MANAGING A CONSORTIUM

- Organize and conduct the first steering committee meeting.
- Summarize networking discussions—agreements and differences of opinion.
- Summarize research and develop a common understanding of the benefits and challenges of simulation education.
- Share lessons learned from others in implementing simulation centers.
- Make recommendations on the roles of committees, task forces, and staff.

■ Agree on the initial vision, mission, and values, or ask a team from the steering committee to make recommendations at the next meeting.

DEVELOPING A STRATEGIC PLAN

■ Meet with the task force to develop a draft of the strategic plan.

■ Ask for input on the region's simulation education environment—trends, opportunities, and threats.

■ Gain agreement on the vision, mission, and values.

■ Share the steering committee's vision, mission, and values.

■ Discuss similarities and differences.

■ Describe the desired future of simulation education in the region.

■ Describe the current state of simulation education in the region.

■ Develop strategies and goals that will move the consortium to the desired future of simulation education in the region.

■ Identify the resources required to meet the strategies and goals.

■ Identify the benefits, outcomes, and measures.

■ Develop a draft of a project plan.

■ Meet with the steering committee to share and finalize the strategic plan.

EVALUATING THE STRATEGIC PLAN

■ Describe to administrators and simulation users the benefits and challenges of developing and using an evaluation plan for achieving the strategic goals.

■ Meet with the steering committee and task force to discuss successful strategies.

■ Define the different aspects of a comprehensive and successful regional simulation education system.

■ Define an evaluation process that would help measure progress toward achieving success—include both short- and long-term goals.

■ Request input from additional key stakeholders and partners.

- Gain approval for the initial evaluation.
- Review progress regularly and redefine annually.
- Provide recognition opportunities.

PLANNING FOR PROFESSIONAL DEVELOPMENT

- Involve steering committee, task force members, and other simulation users in a professional needs assessment data gathering process.
- Involve the same groups in the design of a training matrix that they use in their organizations to track the development of educators and health care professionals in attaining the knowledge and skills of simulation education.
- Provide a variety of professional development opportunities that capture the diversity of learning styles that exist in any large group.
- Evaluate the effectiveness of training and education courses, webinars, workshops, and so on to assure they are meeting the objectives and needs of the participants.
- Provide research opportunities as well as regional and national exposure to simulation education users who have demonstrated initiative and success in their application of simulation.
- Where possible, provide professional continuing education units for participation in the opportunities provided.
- Assist consortium members in providing tools that help them do their work more effectively and efficiently—for example, a regional simulation library.
- Provide exposure to regional and national experts in simulation.
- Remove obstacles in the way of a comprehensive regional simulation professional development program.

IMPLEMENTING THE STRATEGY

- Meet regularly with the steering and professional development committees to report progress on goals.
- Check priorities with steering and professional development committees and provide information on next steps.

- Communicate with all stakeholders through newsletters, Web sites, press releases, and presentations.
- Highlight accomplishments, "islands of excellence," and short-term successes. Pay particular attention to providing a balanced view that acknowledges the accomplishments of all partners.
- Ask for advice and help from others when a project becomes "stuck"—we all have leadership qualities and strengths in specific situations.
- Eliminate barriers through joint problem solving.
- Learn about each partner's environment to appreciate and understand the decisions they make.
- Begin the process of determining which benefits of simulation should be included in our sustainability plan.

ENGAGING IN REFLECTION AND RENEWAL

- Complete a collaboration survey.
- Review results against the strategic plan and evaluate the benefits.
- Discuss lessons learned.
- Scan the environment; look for new trends, opportunities, and threats.
- Review the vision, mission, and values statements—make adjustments after discussion and consensus.
- Take another look at consortium strengths, weaknesses, opportunities, and threats.
- Develop the next iteration of the strategic plan.
- Prioritize the next round of strategies, goals, and action steps.
- Review new resource requirements.

PLANNING FOR SUSTAINABILITY

- Develop a funding and sustainability subcommittee from the steering committee members.
- Review the benefits of the simulation center project.
- Prioritize future work and benefits that the consortium wants to maintain, and transfer or eliminate programs as appropriate.

- Review the new resource requirements.
- Involve the steering committee is scanning for new grants, or other funding sources.
- Update and maintain a grant template that describes the successes of the consortium.
- Build alliances with other groups with similar missions.

FIVE

Developing a Strategy

Every moment spent planning saves three to four in execution.
—Steven G. Haines (1995, p.2)

Good fortune is what happens when opportunity meets with planning.
—Thomas Alva Edison

We will not lie to you: Developing a strategic plan is no one's idea of a good time. It requires time, patience, a willingness to collaborate (there is that word again!), and a big-picture perspective. But putting the effort into the front end of the process will streamline your consortium's work by identifying goals, mapping a route with strategies to reach those goals, and will keep you from straying off course as new opportunities arise. Although it does require work, remember that strategic planning is not an endurance race. With careful preparation, you can develop a framework for your strategic planning process that will help smooth your course over the next 2–3 years.

The strategic development work marks a critical stage in your consortium progress. During this time, your partners may have some of their most vigorous discussions: Deciding the starting and ending points of your work is relatively easy, but agreeing upon the best routes between them can be challenging. Take the time you need: A consortium's ability to integrate planning and action on a continuous basis allows them to become more efficient and effective and produce outstanding results. With the appropriate collaborative spirit and a thoughtful, flexible plan, your consortium can develop working strategies to reach its goals while responding to your partners' needs. Your first steps will be to assess your market and create a needs assessment that captures the details of your educational needs and the ways that simulation technology will address them.

PHASE I: GATHERING INFORMATION

At this point in your process, you have established the foundation of your consortium: The partners have established the initial network, created its governing and organizational structures, and founded collaboration as the theme of your work. You understand roughly where you are and where you want to go. Now, you just need to fine-tune those compass points and plot your journey. The OSA was the first consortium to implement a business model to define its market and inform its planning strategies—a process that the alliance revisits each year (See Exhibit 5.1 for more information on defining a market). A needs assessment scans the current environmental conditions and identifies projected needs that will provide the basis and rationale for your strategic plans. You may also refer to it later in your consortium's life cycle as you develop grant applications, so the work you put in now will pay off later.

EXHIBIT 5.1
Analyzing the Market

Oregon Simulation Alliance
Michael Seropian, MD, and Bonnie Driggers

Each year, the OSA investigates its relevance in the health care market by asking questions like these: Have we done the job we set out to do? What is the market? What groups are ready for simulation? Who needs simulation? Rather than making the argument that simulation adds value, this approach allowed us to focus on where—and how—the market needs us most. Initially, that market was expanding simulation instructor experience in nursing, but its simulation needs have evolved. Over the last several years, the OSA expanded into EMS. The physician market is still evolving. Because the OSA maintained the diversity of its board, with a mix of nurses, physicians, and EMS and allied health professionals, it has remained flexible to react to an ever-changing marketplace.

Developing a Needs Assessment

Remember the original research that gathered general information about simulation education to establish a baseline of knowledge for your consortium? Use it as the basis for the needs assessment. Your strategic planning committee can expand on that work by gathering information on all aspects of simulation. The committee should "triangulate" its research by approaching the topic from different angles: literature review and quantitative and qualitative analyses. In Exhibit 5.2, Mary Lou Brunell of the Florida Center for Nursing describes their approach to the needs assessment.

EXHIBIT 5.2
Scanning the Environment

Florida Center for Nursing
Mary Lou Brunell

In our data-gathering process for "Promoting the Use of Simulation Technology in Florida," a project funded by the Nurse Education Partners Investing in Nursing's Future, we surveyed hospital and nurse education settings, listened to focus groups and interviews, and gained a broader understanding of the policy side of the issue from legislative leaders. We performed a quantitative survey, and I visited simulation centers throughout the state and nation. We also held a think tank early in 2011.

We identified barriers to increasing educational capacity of the current educational system, such as (1) clinical space, (2) a finite number of patients who are willing to work with student nurses, (3) an aging population of nurses who are resistant to new technology or who wish to change jobs, and (4) a changing patient demographic that includes much more home-based care. Simulation stood out as an intriguing, safe, and realistic environment for learning.

The Literature Review

Your literature review will collect, organize, and evaluate the published information about simulation education, including journal articles, books, conference proceedings, and government and corporate reports. For easy interpretation and retrieval on a later date, your review can organize key points into specific categories, such as the following:

■ Environmental factors that others have experienced or considered significant; for example, the geographic location of the partners and how they can work together through several regional simulation centers or one centrally located center
■ Types of simulators and simulation scenarios
■ Potential uses of simulation in postsecondary and continuing education
■ Typical simulated scenarios for medical and surgery specialties
■ Potential user groups of simulation for educational purposes
■ Advantages of clinical simulation
■ Challenges of clinical simulation
■ The administrative and financial investments of running a simulation center
■ Lessons learned from others in planning, completing needs analysis, staffing, program development, training, maintenance, outcomes, funding, sustainability, advantages of collaboration, governance structure, and costs of simulation equipment and implementation

Your literature review provides an overview of the simulation picture in your region. Quantitative and qualitative research will flesh out this picture with specific data.

Quantitative and Qualitative Research

Quantitative data can be efficiently gathered, measured, and analyzed, while allowing generalized results from a sample to a larger population, but may miss contextual detail. Sources of quantitative data include questionnaires, surveys, and structured interviews. Qualitative research techniques, on the other hand, will provide insights into the needs and opinions of a target population. They can help researchers identify key issues for further follow-up. Sources of qualitative data include unstructured interviews and focus group sessions. Interview subjects can include simulation experts; nurse educators; hospital administrators; practicing nurses; consortium center managers, faculty, and staff; industry leaders; nursing students; and recent nurse graduates.

You will use this research process to draw a picture of the current health care environment within the consortium's reach and identify factors and trends that may affect the strategic plan, including the following:

- The demand for health care services
- Shortage of registered nurses and other health care occupations
- The current state of simulation education in their region
- Simulation equipment
- Simulation applications
- Size and demographics of user groups
- The number of nurse educators who need training
- An estimate of costs required to purchase equipment and provide laboratory space, debriefing rooms, and ancillary materials such as audiovisual equipment and simulation supplies
- Current and projected capabilities of simulation education and the future of simulation education in educational institutions and clinical settings that they desire for their region

You will also consider the strengths, weaknesses, opportunities, and threats that exist internally within the consortium and external factors that may have an impact on the strategic plan. Once you have used this information to identify the gap between your current situation and your ultimate goals, you can begin developing key methods to close the gap, such as the following:

- Measures to help track progress of the consortium's work
- Resource requirements to support the plan
- A budget to implement the projects
- A sustainability plan—identification of factors and benefits the consortium members expect

To accomplish the goals of your consortium—to enact the strategic plan—you need to understand which resources are required to produce the desired outputs. In very practical terms, how much is the consortium willing to add resources to planning and implementing a simulation center?

Managing the Workflow: The Reservoir Principle

Information gathering can be a remarkable amount of work—one that even the best planning may not prepare you for. In the early stages of a consortium, you may not have a full understanding of its capacity to handle the workflow. Try to imagine it as a reservoir storing and processing water. Like a reservoir, a controlled system manages the flow effectively. The reservoir principle requires consortium leaders to manage the input and output of work (like water) so not to exceed the capacity of the system at each moment in time. When assuming new activities within the strategic planning process, the reservoir principle provides the following suggestions to help manage the workflow:

- Rather than looking at each task individually, take "big picture" view of the work-cycle trends within your consortium. How fast does an idea mature into an action item? Does an activity (i.e., information gathering) have an ending point, or is it continuous? If the latter, does the level of work fluctuate? Is the work effort required for a single point in time or does it have a repetitive nature (variable)? Do the work outputs deliver what we expected and/or desired?
- Be conservative when accepting new work or projects into the system. Make sure the reservoir can handle this new input.
- Where possible, prioritize work or projects that improve the quality of the system and/or reduce the level of work required, i.e., process improvement initiatives.
- Track the work. If processes or goals overlap, projects may be combined. The best time to make improvements in process is at the design stage.
- Document new ideas, even if they are not immediately achievable. As the strategic planning process continues, the consortium grows in capacity or focus, or the capabilities of simulation increase, some ideas may develop "new legs."

PHASE II: DISCUSSION

Once you have completed your scan of the environment, you can use this information to encourage discussion of strategic choices and decisions. You may decide to use a professional facilitator to manage this dialogue. According to Mary Lou Brunell, the organizers of Florida's Partners Investing in Nursing's Future simulation project think tank found a facilitator incredibly helpful: "We didn't plan to use a facilitator, but we had the funds, thought that expert assistance would be a valuable asset, and so hired a facilitator who did an excellent job. We found that it really helped to have someone with a talent for engaging the audience rather than presenting information to them."

Exhibit 5.3 shows the flow of discussion resulting from the Southeast Indiana Health Care Consortium's regional environmental scan. To organize the discussion, the facilitator grouped the data into categories.

The consortium can keep these key points in mind as they develop their strategic choices of action. That development process includes describing the consortium's vision of simulation education in the future—their goals—as well as the current state of simulation education. By using these descriptions to outline the gap between these two views, the consortium can begin to develop a plan to close it.

EXHIBIT 5.3
Findings From an Environmental Scan

Community/Environment

- The unemployment rate in the region has increased from 4% to 10% in the last three years. Vacancy rates in nursing are currently low due to a weak economy.

  Discussion: As the economy improves, how will that affect turnover and demand for nurses, particularly nursing faculty, because these numbers tend to effect future numbers of nursing graduates? How can our consortium address the educational needs of this changing population?

- The population is aging and the numbers of citizens aged 65 years and older are increasing more than 20%.

  Discussion: How will this affect the health care demand in the near future? What are the health care needs of this increasing population, and how can our consortium help the nursing profession in our region adapt?

Educational Needs/Trends

- There exists a great demand for high-quality clinical sites and experiences.

  Discussion: Can this be improved with the use of clinical simulation? What is the likelihood of the State Board of Nursing organizations increasing the allowable percentage of clinical time through simulation?

- Technological changes increase the demand for higher levels of education for nurses and practitioners.

  Discussion: Are training and educational programs resourced sufficiently to handle the demand? Through simulation centers, can the consortium increase capacity and capability of knowledge and skills? How so?

- Health care professionals increasingly demand an exciting work environment in which they learn and grow through their work assignments and professional development opportunities.

  Discussion: How can simulation technology provide these opportunities?

- The demand for critical thinking skills continues to grow. The confidence of both students and professionals increases with effective simulation learning opportunities and well-executed debriefing sessions (Jeffries, 2007).

  Discussion: How can the consortium provide simulation technology and help develop exercises and scenarios that encourage critical thinking and confidence among nurses?

Simulation Center Needs/Challenges

- Considering the preparation-practice gap, academia and hospitals must work together more closely.

  Discussion: How can the simulation consortium help these two entities collaborate to better prepare nursing students for the realities and challenges of the workplace?

- Some of the challenges that new simulation centers can experience are insufficient space, resources, training, and

technical assistance in the maintenance of equipment and
supporting ongoing operations.

*Discussion: How can the consortium address these challenges
in a comprehensive, fiscally responsible way?*

Envisioning the Future

By now, the task force has a growing collection of resources available to them to complete a vision of the future of simulation for their
consortium, including the following:

- Vision and mission statements
- Core values
- Summary of the research on simulation
- Results of an environmental scan

Using this information, the strategic plan committee's next
action is to complete the plan, detailing how to reach their stated
goals in light of their vision, mission, and core values.

The committee chair can lead a visioning session in one meeting and provide committee members with a summary during a second meeting to gain consensus. Some questions that may be posted
to help task force members write their own visions of the future
include the following:

- What is the purpose of simulation for our consortium?
- Who will use simulation?
- What will be the benefit of simulation for our region?
- How will the plan demonstrate our values?
- What resources need to be available for simulation to work well
  in our region?
- How would we know when success has been achieved?
- What barriers must be overcome?

After each task force member has completed the exercise, the
facilitator can lead the group in dialogue and clarify points for the
group. At the next meeting, the facilitator can provide a summary
for further discussion. Table 5.1 illustrates an example summarizing
a visioning meeting for a regional consortium.

TABLE 5.1

Summary of Consortium Goals and Metrics

SIMULATION GOAL FOR THE CONSORTIUM	OUTCOME METRIC FOR THE REGION
Improve patient safety	Regional metrics show improvement
Improve critical thinking skills of nursing students and new nursing graduates	The region creates a measurement for critical thinking that can be shared and used by all partners
Prepare students for clinical setting experiences	Each regional clinical setting will work with educational partners to prepare a simulation curriculum and experience that prepares students well
Increase number of learning encounters and applications	Greater number of simulation education learning encounters and applications that align with hospital staff education needs
Progress nurses more rapidly through the stages of learning, as described by Benner (2010)	Nurses move rapidly through orientation and become more confident in handling a variety of situations and improve critical thinking skills
Develop a professional development curriculum for all simulation users	A training and education matrix provides multiple options for simulation users to continuously learn
Ensure that each health care partner has the simulation equipment best suited for their desired applications	A needs assessment has been completed and applications identified. A variety of equipment is provided to meet those needs: task trainers; low-, medium-, and high-fidelity simulation equipments; computer-aided instruction; and other blended approaches
Provide technology assistance for all institutions	Each health care partner in the consortium has the technological support to maintain scenario development and maintenance of manikins
Define process improvement for all institutions	Simulation education is seen as a methodology to innovative approaches to process improvement

In this example, the goals have aggregated around resource requirements and outcomes of applying those requirements in simulation education.

DEFINING THE CURRENT STATE OF SIMULATION EDUCATION

Your committee's next steps in this strategic planning process are to take a critical look at the current state of simulation education and complete a SWOT (Strengths, Weaknesses, Opportunities, and Threats) analysis, which identifies and articulates the strengths and weaknesses within an institution, as well as the external opportunities and threats. A SWOT analysis matches the resources and capabilities of the consortium to the external environment.

A facilitator can lead the SWOT analysis process and summarize the findings. It is helpful to explain to task force members the differences between strengths, weaknesses, opportunities, threats, internal assessment, and external environmental factors. Strengths and weaknesses are internal factors focused to the consortium, whereas opportunities and threats are external factors that may impact the consortium. The following list suggests questions to help foment discussion and stimulate creative thoughts:

Strengths
- What are our unique strengths?
- What do we do better than anyone else?
- What resources and skills are we most proud of?
- What positive trends exist in our environment?

Weaknesses
- What skills and resources should we improve?
- What pitfalls should we avoid?
- What skills and resources do we lack?
- What concerns do we have?
- What pressures do we feel?

Opportunities
- What possibilities do we see for our consortium and the future of simulation education?
- Given our assets and resources, what can we accomplish if we work together?

Threats

■ What outside factors could influence us negatively?

■ What outside barriers to success do we see?

Take the time to listen to each participant and collect all of the input. The committee chair can present the aggregate themes in each category at the next meeting. After discussion and reaction to the list, the facilitator can lead the group through a list of priority setting that will show the strength of each theme and help make the list more manageable. Table 5.2 displays an example SWOT analysis completed by consortium members focusing on developing simulation resources or a simulation center.

Key Potential Actions

Immediately after the SWOT analysis and discussion have been covered, the task force can continue with a creative exercise that identifies possible actions that would utilize their strengths and opportunities,

TABLE 5.2
Completed SWOT Analysis

STRENGTHS	WEAKNESSES
1. Magnet Award Status and other awards	1. Decrease in patient safety performance
2. Quality of staff	2. Lack of appropriate staffing levels—quantity and quality
3. Emphasis on education	3. Lack of experience and understanding of clinical simulation
4. Stability of workforce	
5. Relationships between educational institutions and hospitals	4. Generation gap between faculty, staff, and patients
6. Increase in the number of ASN/BSN graduates in the region	

OPPORTUNITIES	THREATS
1. Regional collaboration	1. Complexity of equipment
2. Potential funding sources	2. Low utilization of equipment reported by others
3. Access to simulation training and education	3. Maintain diligence in key processes—curriculum development, scenario development, debriefing, assessment, and evaluation
4. State and national relationships	

and reduce or eliminate weaknesses and threats. The output of the exercise can be placed in "the reservoir" for future consideration. The implementation of the strategic plan may bring opportunities to address some of the actions in the reservoir. Table 5.3 illustrates how a SWOT analysis can help a consortium determine its actions.

TABLE 5.3
SWOT Analysis Output and Action Items

CONCEPTS/THEMES FROM SWOT ANALYSIS	ACTION ITEMS
Emphasis on quality education	Conduct forums where quality techniques and methods are shared with others in the region. For example, at a regular task force group meeting after implementation
Several partners in the consortium have won quality awards	Promote health care partners thorough a web site, newsletter, and press releases. This would require regular scanning of recognition opportunities throughout the region
The relationship between educational institutions and hospitals is good	Develop lesson plans, scenarios, and key learning outcomes and place them in a regional library available to all partners
Consortium over time can be formalized	Report common regional data on measures of interest—vacancy rates, number of learning encounters, success stories, and actions to avoid
Technical expertise in simulations is developed	Contract with a technical consultant to help develop a "train the trainer" capability; track good practices and spread across the region
Concerns about maintenance, warranty, and ongoing costs	Benchmark certain items, e.g., warranties, maintenance costs, etc., with other sites similar to the simulation system you are wanting to implement
Concerns about purchasing equipment beyond capability and use	Have the technical consultant complete a needs assessment of applications needed in the future and make recommendation on equipment purchases

This is a small sample of the kind of actions that understanding strengths, weaknesses, opportunities, and threats can produce. By developing future scenarios on how to use the consortium knowledge in these areas, elements of a strategic plan begin to emerge.

Develop Core Strategies

Armed with the information and analysis performed by the strategic planning committee, the entire consortium can meet to identify 5–7 core strategies. After choosing the core strategies, determine their implementation sequence and the relationship between each of the strategies; i.e., must they be implemented in sequence to each other, or can some be implemented in parallel? Core strategies might include the following:

- Contract with a technical consultant for assistance. This person could educate the steering committee on simulation, work with the task force to develop a project plan, and develop and communicate goals.
- Develop a comprehensive professional development plan for the consortium.
- Complete a project plan including budget, timetable, milestones, and measures of success.

After developing and prioritizing the strategies, present them to your steering committee for approval. Once they have been reviewed and approved, the strategic plan committee can begin the implementation plan.

BEGINNING THE IMPLEMENTATION: THE PROJECT PLAN

Developing a high-level project plan breaks down the elements of your goals and the estimated time to complete them. (For a sample project plan, see Exhibit 5.4.). Exhibit 5.5 describes one consortium's surprising discoveries as they began implementing their plan.

The consortium can develop well-written goals for most major activities that have such measurable characteristics as costs, quality, delivery, customer satisfaction, or any other dimension of performance. Table 5.4 shows some example goal statements corresponding with the activities listed on the sample project plan provided in Exhibit 5.4.

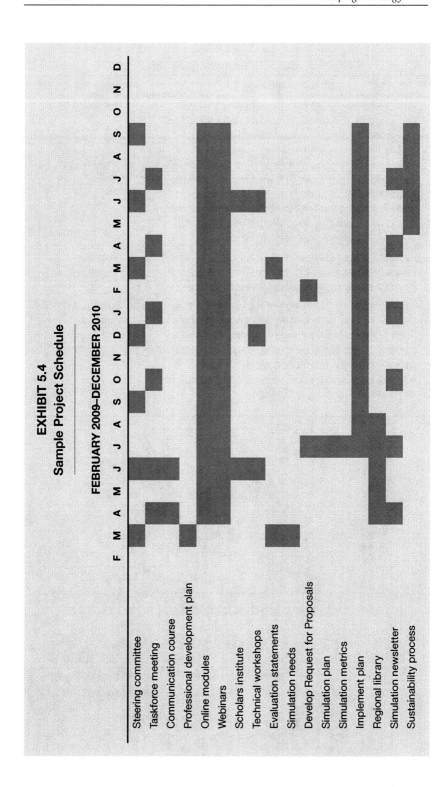

EXHIBIT 5.4

Sample Project Schedule

FEBRUARY 2009–DECEMBER 2010

TABLE 5.4

Sample Goal Statements

GOAL STATEMENT	PROJECT PLAN ITEM
A process for request for appropriations will be designed by the consultant and coordinator and approved by the steering committee. Based on the needs assessment and subsequent interviews and/or conference calls, decisions will be made in two phases: (1) as soon as possible, to fulfill the initial need for equipment, space, and professional development, and (2) a second round of proposals, once the partner organizations have gained experience in simulation.	Develop RFPs
A balanced scorecard of measures will be in place at the regional level. Local measures are encouraged to support the regional level of measures.	Simulation metrics
A sustainability committee will be formed within one year of the end of the initial strategic plan. Their outcomes will provide a summary of the resources and assets within the regional health care community, and suggestions for future funding to extend the benefits of the consortium beyond the original grant period.	Sustainability process

EXHIBIT 5.5

Flexible Plans

Southeast Indiana Health Care Consortium
Dave Galle

During our initial information-gathering phase, we educated our simulation task force on the technology and then asked them to think into the future: what would they like to see, what applications they could imagine using, and how many people they expected to train. We turned that information over to our simulation expert, who held conference calls with each partner to ask them about their needs and goals, and made recommendations on equipment.

Even though we had an expert, we made a strategical decision not to spend all the money right away. We established a basic level of simulation in each location, with the expectation of at least one more round of purchase because the centers did not know what they did not know. Now that they have some familiarity and expertise with it, we can tailor future equipment to their newly discovered needs. And we have found that they are moving away from equipment purchases to ancillary supplies and teaching tools and techniques, maybe a different type of professional development. We are getting some creative ideas at this point, so we think that it was wise to hold back some money and adjust our plans accordingly.

As an example, one consortium group established a goal for the support staff to complete research and evaluation of simulation practices over a three-month period. The group was particularly interested in knowing complete and accurate estimated costs for constructing a simulation laboratory, a control room, and a debriefing room, as well as costs for simulation equipment, audiovisual equipment, and maintenance and warranties. Finally, the consortium explored the advantages and disadvantages of simulation education methodology and the potential benefits of developing it in their region. The steering committee allocated a sufficient amount of budget to support the research activity and set a date for completion.

This example provides some basic goal parameters: the actions to be performed by the support staff, the rationale behind the actions, specific topics or issues to cover, scope of budget, and deadlines. However, within those outlines, the support staff enjoyed a great deal of freedom on *how* to complete the work, such as identifying sources, choosing methods of presenting their findings, or following informational threads that their research uncovered. The goal parameters actually allowed them to display their own initiative and creativity. If developed with high performance standards, goals show clarity and enhance the motivation and interest of the consortium.

Project plans typically cover 1 year—perhaps as many as 2 years, with work defined in broad categories. When executing the strategy, a quarterly examination of goals provides sufficient lead time to organize and complete work. The project plan also reduces duplication of effort: By visually representing goals and activities, the plan makes it easier to synchronize the efforts to achieve them. Integrating work enables more productive effort, thereby reducing the throughput time (the time to complete a given activity).

LESSONS LEARNED

- Managing capacity and demand through the reservoir principle is one of the keys to success.
- Visioning the future and planning strategies is an ongoing process.
- Environmental conditions can change rapidly.
- The same issue can show up as both a strength and a weakness, depending on the "eye of the beholder."
- Although the process may be arduous, strategies tend to emerge easily.

SUMMARY

Although developing the strategic plan can consume a lot of a consortium's time and energy—the entire process may take up to 12–16 hours over three or four meetings—you will find that the work is a worthy investment. Planning ahead does not plot out a rigid course for your consortium to follow; rather, a good plan allows for midcourse corrections as conditions arise or information is uncovered. The Oregon Consortium for Nursing Education, for instance, has re-created its strategic plan a couple of times since the original group came together in 2001: once in 2006–2007 and again in 2011 to address the Institute of Medicine (IOM)'s 2010 Future of Nursing report, consider options for sustainable and permanent funding, and keep abreast of dynamic changes in health care. By and large, investing the creative input of your consortium now will help you see the horizon ahead.

Because most strategic plans cover 2–3 years, the consortium will need to revise the plan, but the time spent establishing the process means that subsequent planning sessions will be much more efficient. Over time, the planning process becomes continuous and seamlessly woven into the work of the consortium.

REFERENCES

Benner, P., Sutphen, M., Leonard, V., & Day, L. (2010). *Educating nursing: A call for radical transformation.* San Francisco, CA: Jossey-Bass.

Haines, S. G. (1995). *Successful strategic planning.* Menlo Park, CA: Crisp.

Jeffries, P. R. (2007). *Simulation in nursing education: From conceptualization to evaluation.* New York, NY: The National League for Nursing.

SUGGESTED READINGS

Costello, S. J. (1994). *Effective performance management.* Burr Ridge, IL: Business One Irwin/Mirror Press.

Mager, R. F. (1984). *Goal analysis* (2nd ed.). Belmont, CA: Pitman Management and Training.

Pfeffer, J., & Sutton, R. I. (2000). *The knowing-doing gap: How smart companies turn knowledge into action.* Boston, MA: Harvard Business School Press.

SIX

Evaluating the Strategic Plan

If you cannot measure it, you cannot improve it.
—Lord Kelvin

Once the strategic plan has been reviewed and approved by the steering committee, your next step will be to develop an evaluation plan to measure the success of the plan outcomes. The fact is the implementation of your strategy tosses a lot of balls into the air: The evaluation plan helps you juggle them. It will help you keep track of their progress, generate data to return to the stakeholders (and to include in future grants), and, if an approach is not working, allow you to change tactics before investing your resources too heavily. Evaluation tools can help the consortium attack the issue from different angles: A balanced scorecard measures progress from various perspectives of achievement, while evaluation statements integrate opinions and input from the partners.

WHY BOTHER?

Establishing goals and measures to evaluate the strategic plan's performance helps the consortium

- discover if performance against goals is improving or declining;
- determine how resources and budget allocations should be made;
- motivate the consortium as it implements the strategic plan;
- promote the consortium's efforts and achievements to others; and
- analyze performance factors and develop strategies for improvement.

ESTABLISHING A BASELINE

Now that your strategic plan is complete, your consortium has defined core strategies and action steps in a project plan that shows completion dates for major activities, as well as identified and allocated required resources over the life of the project. Your next step is to evaluate your position by establishing a performance baseline to measure improvement over the life cycle of the initial 3- to 5-year plan.

The activities outlined in the project plan help the staff support team set strategic goals and performance outcomes or results. Initially, the staff support team may want to think about broad goals. The staff support team might develop the following broad goals from the strategic plan:

- Improve safety and patient care
- Improve critical thinking skills
- Reduce transition time of orientation time
- Increase student or health care providers confidence and competence
- Reduce and/or eliminate medical errors and near misses
- Improve retention rates
- Improve staff communication
- Reduce the cost of the total health care system, e.g., shorter stays, more accurate diagnoses
- Improve efficiency through process improvement
- Reduce liability costs
- Improve NCLEX (National Council Licensure Examination) scores

Broad goals become easier to achieve if you break them down into specific, measurable, and attainable goals that are relevant and are time bound (Doran, 1981). In doing so, consider the following questions:

- Is this a short-term or a long-term goal?
- Is this a single goal or part of a sequence of steps leading to a single, larger outcome?
- Is this a quantitative or qualitative goal?
- Is this a process goal or a result goal?

■ What best measures success of the goal? Cost, quality, delivery, participant satisfaction, or other characteristics?

■ Does the consortium have baseline data (measurements) on the goal?

■ Does each member of the consortium agree on the goals?

■ Is each member of the consortium open to sharing data from their institution?

Use the project plan to track progress and guarantee that the consortium's strategic plan implementation stays on course. Exhibit 6.1 illustrates the balanced scorecard format recommended by Kaplan and Norton (1996). This matrix helps you to develop a broad picture of a goal's successes by assessing them from various perspectives (both financial and nonfinancial) across time.

EXHIBIT 6.1
Format to Organize Short- and Long-Term Goals
(Kaplan & Norton, 1996)

PERSPECTIVE OF SUCCESS	SHORT-TERM SUCCESS	LONG-TERM SUCCESS
Participant satisfaction		
Financial implications		
Staff or personnel		
Process		

This matrix measures the success of a goal over the short and long term by the following four perspectives:

■ *Participant satisfaction.* This category provides feedback on a product's or process's success from the participant's perspective (Kaplan & Norton, 1996). For example, a participant satisfaction goal might be to improve patient care and safety. Other goals may include development of a set of core simulations to orient new nursing graduates; training of all staff educators in the system in designing, implementing, and evaluating using simulations.

■ *Financial implications.* To develop such a large enterprise successfully, the consortium needs to consider and outline its financial implications. Kaplan and Norton (1996) define financial considerations as increasing revenues, improving cost and productivity, enhancing asset utilization, and reducing risk. For example, a financial goal might be to improve efficiency through simulation process improvement. Establishing a new innovation such as a regional simulation center will require operating costs, maintenance, and other resources.

■ *Staff or personnel goal.* Staff development ensures that the simulation pedagogy and implementation is delivered in a quality, effective manner. Kaplan and Norton (1996) define staff or personnel goal as meeting staff needs to provide long-term growth and improvement. For example, a staff goal might be to increase the number of hours of professional development per simulation user. In some cases, this issue may act as a barrier to the integration of simulations into the teaching or learning environment (Jeffries, 2007), because educators may not have the time to spend in professional development and the funding to attend such programs. If educators are not trained in using the pedagogy, then they are less likely to integrate simulations into the program. Educators may lack the knowledge and skill set to conduct simulations in the learning environment.

■ *Process goal.* Organizational progress is driven by analyzing processes and taking actions to improve their results. Kaplan and Norton define a *process goal* as the value proposition that will attract and retain an audience. For example, a process goal might be to improve critical thinking skills among students. This measurement also satisfies the steering committee that processes are meeting participant needs in a cost-effective fashion that utilizes the talents and assets of the organization.

By measuring these perspectives over the short term as well as the long term, the consortium can track the progress of goal achievement:

■ *Success over the short term.* The unit of measurement is relative to the overall time necessary to complete a goal. For example, if a simulation scenario must be developed by the end of the semester, a consortium can measure the success of a short-term goal in days. On the other hand, the short-term success of implementing a segment of a 3-year strategic plan could be measured in months. Short-term success in each perspective (participant satisfaction, financial, staff, and process) helps motivate consortium members towards reaching the long-term goals.

■ *Success over the long term.* Long-term goals should still be realistic and attainable within the 2–5 years that span the typical strategic plan.

Measuring the success of a goal over the short and long terms allows a consortium to maintain momentum, while balancing and tracking its progress by the four perspectives.

In addition to measuring specific project goals, the consortium should perform a system-wide self-evaluation. We will review an evaluation approach, the benefits of its use, the challenges, and the results that specific project goals and an evaluation plan can produce.

SYSTEM-WIDE EVALUATION OF THE CONSORTIUM

A system-wide self-evaluation requires consortium partners to collaborate on a series of evaluation statements, approximately 2–3 months after the strategic plan has been approved. These evaluation statements describe the ideal achievement in a specific area of success for the consortium on a regional level and for each educational and clinical site. Table 6.1 details the benefits of this process.

TABLE 6.1
Benefits of Evaluation Statements

BENEFITS	HOW THE BENEFITS ARE ACCOMPLISHED
Provide a structure to organize implementation of the strategic plan	The evaluation statements describe the consortium's mode of operation over topics such as governance structure, strategic planning process, staffing practices, facilities planning, equipment, safety practices, simulation scenario management, education and training requirements, partnerships and collaboration, and measurements

(continued)

TABLE 6.1

Benefits of Evaluation Statements (*continued*)

BENEFITS	HOW THE BENEFITS ARE ACCOMPLISHED
Provides a common approach to improvement and achievement across different consortium partners	Because the statements help the partners agree on operational practices, they have aligned their intents for results and outcomes
Defines all work processes of the consortium	The evaluation plan typically covers 1 year of activity and is reviewed, refined, and updated to account for changes in the environment, clarify statements of operation that have proven not to be useful as stated, and create newer statements that represent higher levels of achievement
Identifies training and education requirements that are necessary to support effective implementation	Consortium leadership can use evaluation statements to identify the required knowledge and skills to implement the strategy. This process defines training and education as an integral part of achieving success
Supports the achievement of key outcomes and results	For all of the reasons listed previously
Supports the development of a regional, state-wide, or national system while providing local control and accountability	The evaluation statements are written at a high enough level to allow flexibility while allowing local control of the process on how to achieve its intent. This places a premium on writing the evaluation statements clearly enough that they represent simulation excellence
Provides a common language and framework	The consortium agrees on definitions of words and the intent of the evaluation process, which is to continuously improve and draw upon the assets and good practices that evolve through their application
Encourages collaboration teamwork and sharing of good practices	The process of sharing individual evaluations of the entire consortium builds collaboration and discussion. Regional evaluation ensures that the infrastructure exists to support the strategic plan and represents the same level of excellence expected at the partner level. Regional statements may apply to every section of the evaluation plan or just specific ones

These benefits may not apply to all consortia, so a given consortium may need to populate this table differently, based on its strategic plan.

Writing Evaluation Statements

The entire consortium participates in developing the evaluation statements, with the steering committee, the consultant, and the coordinator writing the statements for the regional evaluation with task force member and key stakeholder review and input; the task force members or key stakeholder with each consortium partner have input to the set of statements for the individual sites (this one set of statements applies to all of the sites). The partners can work together to develop evaluation statements for the following nine areas of consortium development:

1. Leadership
2. Strategic planning
3. Participant
4. Staff development
5. Facilities, equipment, and safety
6. Information and technology
7. Simulation practices
8. Partnerships and collaboration
9. Performance results

The following example evaluation statement begins with a broad leadership goal:

Leadership

1.0 A leadership structure provides oversight of governance, strategic planning, and implementation of simulation in health care education in our region.

Progressively specific statements about regional and site leadership follow that high-level statement, as illustrated in the following example:

Leadership—Regional

1.1.1 A regional steering committee meets regularly. The committee includes representatives from all participating educational, hospital, and community leaders in the region.

Additional statements (numbered 1.1.2, 1.1.3, and so on) can clarify or expand the evaluation criteria of regional leadership, such as the role of the task force, the simulation education that the steering committee may receive, the steering committee's advocacy role for simulation, and the committee's role in fund-raising activities. See the following example:

> *Leadership—Individual Sites*
>
> *1.1.2 Each organization has included simulation activity in its strategic plan.*

Additional statements in this section might cover the process of completing the evaluation, each organization's role in sustainability, or funding activities. Using the same approach with the rest of the nine areas of consortium development may yield as many as 80–100 unique statements (including regional and individual sites). In this way, the consortium defines its own statements of excellence.

First-level statements should present goals that are relatively easy to attain, with subsequent levels defining goals that are more difficult to achieve. Note that a few words can impact the degree of difficulty. Breaking the statements into different degrees of attainability allows the consortium members to see and track each element of their success and the effort required to achieve them (Table 6.2).

The evaluation statements define the operational level across the consortium that is consistent with the strategic plan. After levels of accomplishment are achieved (or on an annual basis), the consortium can review, re-evaluate, and rewrite statements if necessary. As you develop your evaluation process, remember that

- it is within the consortium's control and responsibility to describe what simulation excellence is for them at a specific point in time;
- working across sites and levels builds a consensus that pays dividends in many ways. For example, collaboration develops trust in strong and reliable ways, while building strengths, eliminating weaknesses, exploiting opportunities, and removing threats effectively.

See Table 6.3 for examples of additional high-level statements for remaining key topics.

Keep in mind that region- and site-specific evaluation statements follow these eight high-level evaluation statements. The power of this evaluation tool lies in its multilevel approach to define, design,

TABLE 6.2

Degrees of Difficulty in Evaluation Statements

LEVEL OF DIFFICULTY	EVALUATION GOAL STATEMENT
First level (low difficulty)	A regional steering committee is established
Second level (intermediate difficulty)	A regional steering committee meets at least quarterly
Third level (high difficulty)	A regional steering committee meets at least quarterly. A representative from each consortium partner serves on the steering committee

TABLE 6.3

Sample High-Level Evaluation Statements

KEY TOPICS	HIGH-LEVEL EVALUATION STATEMENTS
2.0 Strategic planning	A strategic plan is in place that covers simulation activity and describes the actions to be taken
3.0 Staffing development	Personnel are selected, trained, and developed in simulation practices
4.0 Facilities, equipment, safety, and environment	Each organization has designed space for simulation activity and equipment to meet its education needs
5.0 Information and technology	Each site has the technology required to produce effective simulation education scenarios and share in debriefing sessions
6.0 Simulation practice management	Processes are documented to evaluate the design, assessment, evaluation, and guided reflection of simulation scenarios
7.0 Performance, outcomes, and results	Faculty and staff are trained in setting goals, coaching techniques, and identifying developmental opportunities. An environment of continuous improvement helps faculty to meet learning goals
8.0 Partnerships and collaboration	Partnerships and teams increase the effectiveness of the regional learning system in simulation health care education

maintain, and improve. With each statement level increasing in difficulty, the process outlines how significant accomplishments can be made, sustained, and improved. Exhibit 6.2 provides a sample section of this evaluation statement format.

We recommend that the consortium review progress on the evaluation statements each year, removing statements that are no longer useful and adding relevant ones as appropriate.

EXHIBIT 6.2
Sample Strategic Plan Evaluation Statements

Leadership

1.0 A leadership structure provides oversight of governance, strategic planning, and implementation of simulation in health care education in our region.

Leadership—Regional

1.0.1 A regional steering committee meets regularly. The committee includes representatives from all participating educational, hospital, and community leaders in the region.

1.0.2 A regional task force with participation from all consortium partners meets regularly to discuss technical issues related to the implementation of simulation in their organizations.

1.0.3 An educational presentation and materials have been developed and presented to key stakeholders in the region.

Leadership—Individual Sites

1.1.1 Each organization includes simulation activity in its strategic plan.

1.1.2 Each organization has identified personnel to provide for scenario development, scheduling, maintenance, and technical oversight.

1.1.3 Each organization completed an annual evaluation of simulation practices against baseline measures developed at the time of the strategic plan.

Strategic Planning

2.0 A strategic plan that covers simulation activity is described, as well as actions to be taken.

Strategic Planning—Regional

2.0.1 A project plan for the strategic plan time period shows the flow and timing of activities to achieve the overall plan.

Strategic Planning—Individual Sites

2.1.1 Each organization completes a needs assessment to determine the simulation curriculum for the strategic plan period.

2.1.2 Each organization collects and reviews annual data related to simulation laboratory utilization and key measures that support the strategic plan and goals.

Sharing Good Practices Through Self-Evaluation

We can sometimes fail to recognize our own good practices—the actions that provide results in line with the consortium's mission, vision, and core values—simply because they seem to be obvious behaviors or approaches. (See Exhibit 6.3 for background on the OCNE's evaluation strategies.) Luckily, the support staff managing regional consortia have a birds-eye view of good practices developed at various sites; they can help the sites in presenting these exemplar performances to the consortium, detailing how they ensured results and outcomes of specific statements. The coordinator and consultant can also highlight good practices by focusing on how successful results have been achieved.

A systematic method for contributing good practices asks each leader to share their evaluation statements with the consortium on a specific area of organizational development (leadership, strategic planning, staffing, and so on). This information-sharing experience provides participants with the opportunity to ask questions on specific evaluation statements and results.

The leadership can also encourage partners to review and share good practices by assigning a point value to the difficulty of each evaluation statement. For example, an easily achievable statement

EXHIBIT 6.3
Strategic Plan: A Flexible Response to the Environment

Simulation and Clinical Learning Center at the OHSU and OCNE
Paula Gubrud-Howe

It took us about a year to create the first strategic plan, which we re-evaluated in 2006–2007. We will be updating it again in the Spring of 2011, in part because of the Institute of Medicine's 2010 Future of Nursing report demanding better, seamless advanced education to prepare nurses to lead change and advance health. But there are two other major reasons for updating our strategic plan: (a) We are nearly out of grant funding and have not established sustainable and permanent funding and (b) the still-emerging results from ongoing data collection. We received a Robert Wood Johnson Foundation grant that allowed us to create several instruments that measure "fidelity" to our agreements. We have been collecting data for 2–3 years and will be using the data and analysis to inform our strategic planning.

OCNE has moved from an era of start-up and development to creating focused actions that will create a permanent sustainable organization. In keeping with the dynamic nature of change in health care, OCNE leaders are reviewing and revising the consortium's strategic plan. The essential elements that define the benefits of the collaboration have been identified through a comprehensive evaluation study funded by the Robert Wood Johnson Foundation. Consequently, the strategic plan is being adapted to sustain OCNE "best practices" and to accommodate new and redefined strategic goals and initiatives. OCNE partners overwhelmingly credit the consortium with improved quality and continued innovation in curriculum. All member schools are committed to continued participation in OCNE as a means to leverage resources. Our commitment to collaboration has indeed improved the quality and accessibility of nursing education, which ultimately impacts the health of Oregonians in every corner of our state.

may have a value of one point, a difficult statement may have two points, and a very difficult statement may have three points. After the consortium agrees on the statements and degrees of difficulty, each organization can complete a self-evaluation. The support staff can facilitate meaningful comparisons by presenting spreadsheets that show the point scoring for each of the statements. Analyzing the data allows the consortium to compare overall scores and assess each section of the evaluation on its own merit. For example, leadership may have a percentage score for the consortium of 74%; strategic planning may have a score of 68%; staffing 83%; facilities, equipment safety, and environment a score of 62%; and so on. Variations in specific statement scores can also be analyzed. When using this approach, meaningful dialogue can take place and good practices shared, as each site discusses differences of the individual statements.

As the consortium's collaboration grows, evaluation statements will advance to higher levels of difficulty and members will share their good practices more frequently. In this manner, the overall evaluation scores of the consortium tend to rise along with the complexity of its work. This synergy of group collaboration works to improve the overall performance of the consortium. This process also helps to identify the knowledge and skills needed by consortium members; this information can be funneled into a formal professional development plan.

LESSONS LEARNED

- All partners within the consortium must be involved in the development of evaluation statements. If the statements become the sole responsibility of the steering committee, they will be less meaningful and more difficult to attain.
- Baseline evaluation and analysis of results clarifies the consortium's action steps.
- By and large, organizations take responsibility for increasing the level of difficulty of evaluation statements.
- Correlating the evaluation results to the balanced scorecard measures provides the feedback necessary to assure alignment of actions to high-level goals.

■   Project plans are closely linked to organization goals and outcomes, which motivates volunteers and improves overall performance.

SUMMARY

By developing an evaluation process for the strategic plan and goals, your consortium will be able to measure success and set direction for the consortium. A comprehensive evaluation plan for the simulation consortium model consists of two parts: (a) the balanced scorecard of short- and long-term performance measures, covering satisfaction, financial considerations, staff development, and process improvement and (b) a set of evaluation statements and criteria that are updated on an annual basis and represent simulation excellence. Both tools provide valuable data from different perspectives that consortia can use to ensure that their work remains relevant and focused over several years.

REFERENCES

Doran, G. T. (1981). There's a S.M.A.R.T. way to write management goals and objectives. *Management Review, 70,* 35–36.

Jeffries, P. R. (2007). *Simulation in nursing education: From conceptualization to evaluation.* New York, NY: The National League for Nursing.

Kaplan, R. S., & Norton, D. P. (1996). *The balanced scorecard: Translating strategy into action.* Boston, MA: Harvard Business School Press.

Lord Kelvin. (1883). From "Electrical Units of Measurement," a lecture delivered at the Institution of Civil Engineers, London (May 3, 1883). *Popular Lectures and Addresses* (1889) Vol. 1, 73. Quoted in American Association for the Advancement of Science, *Science 19,* 127.

SEVEN

Planning for Professional Development

Develop a passion for learning. If you do, you will never cease to grow.
  —Anthony J. D'Angelo

Many of the steps in this simulation consortium model
concern the high-level effort of building a consortium, i.e.,
activities like strategy and governance development make sure
that the consortium *runs*. This chapter focuses on developing the
actual work of the consortium: providing quality, cost-effective
simulation technology, and education to both practicing nurses
and nursing students. A large part of that initiative lies in professional development, or building a framework to "train the
trainer."

In a simulation consortium, professional development ensures
that simulation users—nurse educators, faculty, instructors, or
anyone who uses simulation in their job—acquire the training and
knowledge to develop, implement, and evaluate simulation scenarios. We provide one method of designing this educational plan, but
many others exist.

ANTICIPATING CHALLENGES

As with any initiative, challenges to designing and implementing a
professional development plan exist. Preparing for them at the start
will help you resolve them quickly, so you can return to the work
at hand: providing simulation education. Table 7.1 outlines some of
these challenges.

TABLE 7.1
Challenges to Professional Development

CHALLENGE	RESPONSE
Employees are "too busy" to dedicate time to simulation education	Simulation education *is* their job. If employees are not trained in simulation techniques, processes, and procedures, they will not be able to perform the jobs—which will ultimately compromise patient quality and safety standards
	Consortium partners must be willing to advocate on behalf of simulation education. Create a few "talking points" detailing the advantages of simulation education
	Less time-consuming learning options, such as webinars, can be taken at home or during work breaks
Knowledge, skills, and abilities for simulation excellence have not been organized to be relevant to current work and strategies	Include personal development objectives in the career trajectory plans and support them with time to learn while on the job
Many people expect education to be delivered via a dry lecture or conference	By design, professional development in simulation education includes engaging, hands-on instruction, often in a group setting that enables participants to share experiences and ideas. Technological and pedagogical advances have also introduced alternative learning methods, including webinars, online training modules, Web site forums
The return on investment for training and education is difficult to quantify	By connecting performance development goals and objectives with individual work plans (including professional development plans), educational outcomes can be tracked with the work goals and objectives of both the organization and individual
	The professional development matrix can help evaluate the capability and capacity of simulation users and support teams throughout the consortium, as well as its organizational partners

ASCERTAINING SPECIFIC LEARNING NEEDS

Remember the evaluation statements your consortium developed to assess the strategic plan? They will come in handy again as you create your professional development matrix. By reviewing the evaluation goals and direction, the consortium can derive the learning needs of its audience. The following list provides ten steps to designing a professional development plan:

1. Analyze evaluation statements to identify potential learning needs.
2. Identify positions in the consortium that may have these learning needs.
3. Develop a matrix that visually breaks out the learners' positions and learning activities.
4. Evaluate each of the activities to determine learning resources available.
5. Provide a variety of learning resources to accommodate diverse learning styles.
6. Determine the specific learning needs of each person in each identified position in need of education.
7. Schedule time for consortium members to learn relevant KSAs (Knowledge, Skills, and Abilities) for their work.
8. Include the development activities in the individuals' work plans.
9. Monitor progress and provide recognition when goals are met.
10. Reinforce learning to application.

Identifying Education and Training Topics

The following offers several education and training topics that you may find during your analysis:

- Simulation awareness
- Scenario design and development
- Debriefing strategies
- Facilitation
- Goal-setting techniques
- Coaching strategies

- Feedback methods
- Personal development
- Strategic planning ideas
- Six sigma and lean techniques
- Curriculum development
- Course scheduling methods
- Data analysis
- Teamwork

Of course, this list is not conclusive, but it does provide potential training areas for your consortium members.

Creating a Simulation Education and Training Matrix

Once you have identified educational topics and positions in need of training, the consortium can develop a simulation and training matrix that shows the knowledge, skills, and abilities required for each position. Table 7.2 illustrates an example of a completed simulation and training matrix. The X populating the cells denotes a topic that the corresponding position needs to learn. As the learner achieves that goal, the X can be changed to a C, for completion.

Of course, this matrix is just a sample. The number and type of positions or roles may differ in your version. The matrix will change over time, as people grow into their professional development. For instance, a trained simulation user will have different learning needs than a first-timer. The number of education and training topics will likely increase, especially after specific simulation scenarios are identified.

Note that the matrix illustrates the educational needs and their achievement; it does not show the type (hands-on or didactic) or quality of the learning that took place, or how that learning was assessed as successful (say, through testing). The consortium itself defines the quality of each education and training topic. During the training, competency testing of the knowledge and skills in developing and implementing simulations can be built into the workshops and programs. All participants in the training need to be aware of the competencies that would be tested, e.g., how to conduct an effective debriefing.

This matrix depicts a consortium overview of education and training requirements and the status of completion. Over time, a key measurement of consortium success in training and education is the percent of achievement of the entire matrix.

TABLE 7.2
Simulation Education and Training Matrix

	STEERING COMMITTEE	SIMULATION USER	TECHNOLOGY SPECIALIST	REGIONAL COORDINATOR	HUMAN RESOURCES	STUDENT
Leadership						
Simulation awareness	x	x	x	x	x	x
Strategic planning						
Strategic planning	x	x		x		
Evaluation statements		x		x		
Human resources						
Job descriptions					x	
Goal setting		x				
Coaching		x				
Providing feedback		x				
Personal development		x				
Working in teams		x				
Information technology						
Programming			x			
Audio visual systems			x			

(continued)

TABLE 7.2
Simulation Education and Training Matrix (*continued*)

	STEERING COMMITTEE	SIMULATION USER	TECHNOLOGY SPECIALIST	REGIONAL COORDINATOR	HUMAN RESOURCES	STUDENT
Simulation practices						
Design and developing simulations		X		X		
Debriefing and guided reflection		X		X		
Guidelines for simulation research		X		X		
Teaching and learning strategies		X		X		
Integrating concepts into simulations		X		X		
Evaluation of simulations		X		X		
Maximizing realism		X		X		
Designing a simulation center		X		X		
Developing faculty		X		X		
Specific simulation scenarios		X				X
Continuous improvement						
Six sigma or lean		X		X		
hardwiring excellence		X		X		
Administration						
Scheduling		X		X		
Data analysis			X	X		

CREATING A COMPREHENSIVE PLAN

The consortium must develop a comprehensive plan to provide the training and education outlined by the matrix. But simulation education requires different approaches from traditional learning. Simulation students learn by participation, observation, and debriefing, rather than through didactic methods. To address this issue, KT Waxman has incorporated Benner's framework into the Bay Area Simulation Collaborative's (BASC) professional development. The BASC plan, which catalogues learners into the stages of novice, advanced beginner, competent, proficient, and expert, ultimately aims to develop students into qualified instructors to teach others. For more information about the BASC plan, see Exhibit 7.1.

EXHIBIT 7.1
Simulation Education: Novice to Trainer

Bay Area Simulation Collaborative
KT Waxman

Our biggest discovery has been that simulation education is not about the technology—it is about the methodology. Most of our faculty and hospital educators were novices at simulation, so we developed initial training at the basic level, covering the concepts, a little technology, the whole pedagogy of simulation, including scenarios and debriefing. They progress through the five levels of the Benner's framework (including an apprentice program), to eventually become our trainers for each region in California. So far, we have trained about 500 in the Bay Area, and Southern California has trained about 200 using our model. We have standardized our model, but it does not present a cookie-cutter approach. The goal is to provide the tools and education so that our learners can implement the education in their own facilities.

Once the consortium has developed a plan outline, it can begin considering the variety of resources and diverse learning methods that will address different stakeholders' learning styles and educational needs. Debi Sampsel, a consortium leader from Wright State University, develops different approaches for different categories of learners. "The science and art behind the activity have to be developmentally appropriate for students to derive value from the technology. For example, we tailor the types of simulation encounters for high school students versus college students. Likewise, the way we use simulation education to bridge new nursing graduates to employment differs from the way we use it for advanced practitioners, faculty, or managers. We develop different simulation tracks so that students can learn to take care of a patient based on their comfort, confidence, and competency levels. As faculty or other continuing educators use simulation to teach, they gain insight into the end users' needs and receptivity. Faculty and health care leaders can improve quality and delivery of care metrics by incorporating simulation into existing educational structures through reengineering the approaches."

One resource to consider for simulation education development is *Simulation in nursing education: From conceptualization to evaluation* (Jeffries, 2007). The book, among the first of its kind for nurse educators, shares the learning experiences of a group of simulation educators over the course of a 3-year multisite project on the use of simulation in nursing education.

Educational conferences for health care professionals offer sessions specifically targeted toward simulation development, implementation, and research. Today, most vendors that sell human patient simulators offer conferences and training for their customers on a regular basis. National organizations offer annual teaching summits or conferences that include sessions on simulation development and implementation or other focused areas of professional development at different geographic locations throughout the year. In addition, different academic institutions are now offering annual workshops to train educators in using the simulation pedagogy, with graduate courses now being available for nurse educators to learn more about the experiential simulation teaching strategy. Considerations for the consortium leaders would include offering financial support for selected educators from the consortium partners to attend the external conferences and workshops.

> *Workshops.* The consortium can offer workshops led by simulation experts and demonstrations presented by simulation vendors, as well as identify state, regional, and national nursing association conferences that provide concurrent sessions led by faculty and practitioners.
>
> *Webinars.* Webinars provide a cost-effective option for regional and state consortia. They typically present information through audiovisual media, can gather information on educational needs through online surveys, and offer a convenient mode of education for the participants. If the consortium has access to a simulation expert, it can contract with the vendor to prepare and design its own webinars. Some vendors offer webinar packages that allow up to 100 participants at a time.

In addition, the National League for Nursing offers online courses in simulation that address different learning needs through lecture, video, and a variety of simulation examples. Each module tests participants and provides a certificate of completion. Individual simulation users can take the courses for continuing education credit; if several faculties and schools want to pool resources, they can obtain a year-long site license for multiple users.

> *Internal resources.* The consortium members can also serve as excellent educational resources. Consortia can develop regional conferences or meetings to present information, create online bulletin boards to encourage the discussion and the sharing of ideas, or facilitate one-on-one training.

Your consortium can implement its professional development plan in numerous ways, but the process requires an innovative approach that considers the specific requirements of this relatively new mode of education. See Exhibits 7.2 and 7.3 for some innovative ideas implemented by the Living Laboratory Smart Technology House at Wright State University and The Simulation Center at Fairbanks Hall.

EXHIBIT 7.2
Interprofessional Learning

Living Laboratory Smart Technology House, a Wright State University, Sinclair Community College, Premier Health Partners, and Graceworks Lutheran Services Funded Community Collaboration
Debi Sampsel

In its first year, our professional development program has seen a lot of interprofessional collaboration from doctors, nursing students, social work students, engineering students, technical students, even business students. We love it! It is enlightening and fun, and it is exactly what we need in health care—for all of the people that are touching the lives of the patients to educate themselves together, in this interactive way. It not only improves relationships, it provides various perspectives to address the complexities of care. For instance, social work students developed case histories and profiles for our simulator family members that include grounded experiences that those cohorts would have experienced in life. They created altered family dynamics that incorporated cultural diversity and non-nuclear structures. We are building a wonderful brain trust.

EXHIBIT 7.3
Preparing for Change

The Simulation Center at Fairbanks Hall
Scott A. Engum, MD

During the early phases of construction, we recognized that we had very few individuals on campus who were equipped to carry out our simulation efforts. We subsequently established an Interdisciplinary Simulation Academy to provide training and initiate a sense of community and collaboration. We invited simulation expert Michael Seropian to introduce us to concepts, best practices, and techniques in simulation, and we then transitioned small groups to simulation scenario case development.

Initially, the Interdisciplinary Simulation Academy served a couple of purposes: to create a cohesive team among the interdisciplinary members of three entities and to learn about such issues as the simulation technology, building cases, and developing evaluations. After the center was open for a year, we discovered that advancing that group has been a challenge because of varying schedules, hours, and hectic schedules of participants. The academy continues to function as a journal club to promote collaboration, knowledge, skills, and attitude advancement. It is our hope to increase the collaborative opportunities and maintain the sense of community among all members.

MEASURING PROFESSIONAL DEVELOPMENT INITIATIVES

Beyond measuring the number of training hours, a number of evaluation methods exist to assess the quality and success of simulation education. Workshop and webinar evaluations, surveys, and the number of continuing education credits achieved all provide well-trodden ways to ensure the quality of your professional development work. There are evaluation tools that can be used to measure competencies, such as the DASH tool (2000) to measure effective debriefing, or the collaboration scale to measure teamwork (Reese, Jeffries, & Engum, 2010). Kirkpatrick's model (1998) can be utilized to measure Kirkpatrick's four-level training evaluation that provides an evaluation methodology for judging training programs. The four levels of evaluation consist of the following: (1) reaction, or how the learners react to the learning process; (2) learning, or the extent to which the learners gain knowledge and skills; (3) behavior, or the capability to perform learned skills while on the job; and (4) results, or the impact of the training program, on areas such as patient safety.

The hierarchical specification of the model implies a natural order for the importance of validation research.

There are also informal measures of success. Consortium leaders reported receiving thank-you letters and other feedback from students who enjoyed their experiences, conducting interviews with faculty on improvement strategies, and getting called back for repeat engagements or getting workshops booked through word of mouth. Document everything, and show it to your advisory committees as proof of your accomplishments.

LESSONS LEARNED

- Education is a continuous process.
- If a student hits a wall in the learning process, try summarizing the work up to that point. This activity can crystallize the information learned and open the mind for continued learning.
- Just-in time-training is essential. If training is provided too early, the context may not be developed enough to allow learning to take hold. A variety of learning opportunities maintain motivation without overwhelming the simulation learners.

We all are teachers and all learners. Sharing with each other develops a common pool of knowledge.

SUMMARY

Professional development sets the cornerstone of your consortium's work: to advance simulation education for the benefit of patient care. To achieve this goal, the consortium requires a comprehensive, well-considered plan that includes an assessment of learning needs, the thoughtful implementation of diverse programs, and a method or tool to evaluate the initiative's success. By assessing, recognizing, and organizing learning opportunities for its members, the consortium continues to build an organizational culture that will support continuous improvement and learning.

REFERENCES

Jeffries, P. R. (2007). *Simulations in nursing education: From conceptualization to evaluation.* New York, NY: National League for Nursing.

Kirkpatrick, D. L. (1998). *Evaluating training programs: The four levels* (2nd ed.). San Francisco, CA: Berrett-Koehler.

Reese, C., Jeffries, P., & Engum, S. (2010). Learning together: Using simulations to develop nursing and medical student collaboration. *Nursing Education Perspectives, 31*(1), 33–38.

Waxman, K. T., & Telles, C. L. (2009). The use of Benner's framework in high-fidelity simulation faculty development: The Bay Area Simulation Collaborative model. *Clinical Simulation in Nursing, 5,* 231–235.

SUGGESTED READINGS

Baxendale, B., & Buttery, A. (2006). Faculty development for simulation-based education and training programmes. Can a national standard be created in the UK? *Simulation in Healthcare: The Journal of Society for Simulation in Healthcare, 1*(2), 116.

Jeffries, P. R. (2008). Getting in S.T.E.P. with simulations: Simulations take educator preparation. *Nursing Education Perspectives, 29*(2), 70–73.

Jeffries, P. R., McNelis, A. M., & Wheeler, C. A. (invited - 2008). Simulation as a vehicle for enhancing collaborative practice models. *Critical Care Nursing Clinics of North America, 20*(4), 471–480.

Lambton, J. (2008). Integrating simulation into a pediatric nursing curriculum: A 25% solution? *Simulation in Healthcare: The Journal of the Society for Simulation in Healthcare, 3*(1), 53–57.

Seropian, M. A. (2004). An approach to simulation program development. *Journal of Nursing Education, 43,* 170–174.

Seropian, M., & Driggers, B. (2005). *The Oregon simulation readiness assessment – evaluating the initial steps of the Oregon simulation implementation model.* Des Plaines, IA: The Society of Critical Care Medicine.

Simon, R., & Raemer, D. B. (2009). *Debriefing assessment for simulation in healthcare.* Cambridge, MA: Center for Medical Simulation.

Simulation Innovative Resource Center (SIRC). Retrieved February 11, 2011, from http://sirc.nln.org/

EIGHT

Implementing the Strategy

To know what people really think, pay regard to what they do, rather than what they say.
—René Descartes

The strategic plan has been completed. It is now time to move on to implementation. Starting this step is like progressing from planning a family road trip to getting in the car. You and the family have selected a location, developed a budget, and made reservations for hotel accommodations at your destination. There will be challenges along the way and unexpected side trips, but you know that if you are adaptable and stay focused on your destination, you will achieve your goals, strengthen your relationships, and even learn a few things. In this chapter, we will review setting goals, developing implementation strategies, responding to challenges, and reporting results and outcomes to keep the consortium apprised of its progress and achievements.

PUTTING A STAKE IN THE GROUND

A consortium is a complex organism, with each system depending on the others. The process of implementation begins by examining the consortium's work organically, with an eye to the goals, desired outcomes, and investment of labor. For example, the consortium can review the activities for its first quarter of implementation with the following questions in mind:

How do the work of different committees align? Make sure that all committees communicate regularly to maintain synchronization, and adjust your project plan to avoid workflow bottlenecks. For instance, because the outcome of steering committee meetings impacts the work of the professional development committee, steering committee meetings should be scheduled first.

How do the perspectives of different committees complement or conflict with each other? Be aware of various perspectives among the committees and ensure that the consortium continues to pursue these opposite but important agendas. For instance, the steering committee takes a global interest in the benefits and challenges of simulation education throughout the region, whereas the professional development group is concerned with the practical challenges of implementing simulation education and its benefits to daily nursing practice. Although different, both are equally important to the business of the consortium and deserve equal support.

What are our practical needs for the next several months? The professional development committee, for instance, will need to consult with the technical consultant to define the equipment each site requires. One goal for the first quarter might be to determine, prioritize, and define the number of students and/or healthcare professionals who need to receive simulation training. To achieve this goal, the committee will need to hold discussions with each partner, using a standard equipment order template and set of questions to collect information on their simulation needs. Determining these needs may take longer than you assume.

How can we break down the workflow into manageable pieces? To begin learning about the operational aspects of simulation, the professional development group will need focus on the types of applications needed, the equipment required, education on simulation scenario development, debriefing, building a library of scenarios, finding or creating space, developing administrative procedures, and so on. No matter how prepared you think you are, you will be surprised at how long each of these requirements will take to consider or complete. The committee needs to sequence each of these activities into a workflow.

How can we plan forward? Good planning creates a domino effect: Typically, each goal you "topple" during a quarter should provide weight and momentum for "toppling" goals during the following quarter. So, evaluating each site's practical needs in the first quarter sets up the creation of the professional development plan in the second quarter. The professional development committee must begin its preparations for designing and/or purchasing educational modules during the first quarter.

The twelve weeks in a quarter sound like a long time, but it goes by quickly. Your coordinator(s) and consultant will perform most of the front-end work in the first quarter, but the rest of the consortium will take on a heavier workload during the following quarters. Despite your best planning and synchronization of effort, unforeseen delays will arise and push back the schedule. Work will accumulate over time, placing stress on the system. But do not forget that your partners have volunteered their time and that they have paid jobs to do, as well as consortium work. Keep an eye on your project plan, trust your collaborators, accept that work will pile up, communicate delays, and practice patience and compassion. The work *will* get done.

Planning for accomplishment also requires planning for challenges to the work. Let's take a look at some of the barriers to large-scale project implementation, and how to manage them before they impact the consortium's ability to produce effective outcomes.

CHALLENGES TO IMPLEMENTATION

Managing implementation in both the short term and long term is not without its difficulties. Problems arise, motivation wanes, and people get stressed. But knowing about the roadblocks and potholes means that you can swerve around them—or at least reduce damage to the vehicle.

Lack of Defining Purpose

When any organization fails to keep its purpose in sharp focus, it loses momentum. Members lose faith in the value of their work, become resentful of their responsibilities, and disengage from the consortium. The consortium's unifying framework breaks down. For instance, occasionally simulation center partners do not understand how their work supports each other—a misconception that returns the consortium to "building functional silos," rather than collaborating in a cohesive way that shows clear benefits to all.

Hopefully, if your consortium has crafted strong mission, vision, and values statements, they can provide a road back to your purpose. By asking high-level questions that clearly connect your consortium's activities with these statements, you can inspire your consortium members' return to commitment. Such questions include the following:

- What is the value of our consortium? What are we trying to accomplish that no one else is? How do we impact patient care as well as the nursing profession?
- How does a specific activity move us closer to our mission and goals? Are there different directions available to us that might be more in line with our mission and goals?

By asking questions and working through answers, we can recontextualize the consortium's work, make it "real," and remind our partners of its value in patient care. In addition, take the time to strengthen relationships between partners, even if it is a small meeting over coffee or simple collaborative projects or team-building exercises. Even with volunteer work, people can get mired in the details of the job and forget the good feelings that come with connecting with others. When the going gets tough, we can all serve as cheerleaders for each other.

Organizational or Cultural Differences

Each partner has its own assets, liabilities, norms, governance structure, and politics that define its organizational culture. For example, academic partners and clinical partners tend to focus on goals and measures of success quite differently. In the early part of the consortium relationship, these variances can become readily apparent. It can become easily apparent of these differences.

Collaboration requires patience and empathy. Understanding the reasons behind your partners' different approaches and goals will neutralize the threat and may highlight the strengths and value they bring to the overall work of the consortium. Not everyone will be adept at these skills, so provide opportunities for discussion to ensure that each partner can articulate the rationale behind their decisions.

Communication

Occasionally, an organization can grow too large for productivity, particularly in the area of communication. The demand for communication exceeds our capacity to respond. Lack of response or miscommunication results in mistakes, which effects implementation. Take steps, such as the following, to ensure that your communication plan grows with your consortium while reinforcing effective communication patterns and reducing those that impede progress:

- Build e-mail distribution lists for specific committees
- Document and distribute the minutes of key meetings
- Prioritize e-mails that require response
- Develop a consortium Web site that is continuously refreshed with news items, events, and information. Track hits to your site as one measurement of your communication efforts
- Develop newsletters to keep stakeholders informed of your consortium's initiatives
- Plan forums for face-to-face interaction and networking
- Commit to frequent communication with key stakeholders. Track the frequency of your communication as a reminder to stay in touch regularly
- Work closely with local and regional newspapers or other publications to keep them informed of your consortium's initiatives. Distribute press releases or special interest stories to advance awareness and interest in simulation education

Despite your best efforts, miscommunication will occur. Acknowledge it immediately, understand how it occurred, and take action to fix it. (See Exhibit 8.1 for Mary Lou Brunell's ideas for communication activities.) Stakeholders understand that even the best systems occasionally break down in small ways; they *do not* understand apathy or failure to respond.

Project Creep

Most of the time, new directions and possibilities indicate healthy organizational growth. Other times, we become entrenched in "project creep"—activities that do not forward our goals. As the

EXHIBIT 8.1
The Web of Communication

Florida Center for Nursing
Mary Lou Brunell

We have a dedicated Web page on the Florida Center for Nursing Web site where I put a lot of our communications, including executive summaries. All of that is open to the public. We have routine communication through our LISTSERV and e-mail distribution lists. We also complete a monthly survey to track who everyone talks to, how often, and what about. The application generates spider graphs to show the huge volume of communication, and if there are gaps in our communication plan, we will be able to spot them. Out grant includes an expectation that we will evaluate communication and collaboration, so theoretically, we could also use the graphs to demonstrate the level of involvement and activity in our organization on this issue.

consortium expands, responsibilities grow more diffuse, and communications systems develop complexity, work will occasionally spiral off into unproductive areas, unnoticed and unchecked. If you suspect project creep, halt and evaluate the work in light of the organization's mission, vision, and values. The following list outlines more strategies for minimizing project creep:

1. Develop a disciplined approach to your work. Test pilot projects or initial steps before committing to a broad action that may, not meet your consortium's goals. Pilot projects provide a safety net and experimental way to evaluate the results or nuances of action steps before beginning a large-scale effort.
2. Brainstorming sessions are great, creative ways to generate new ideas, but do not stop there. Continue your brainstorming to consider resources and methods of implementation. Doing so can weed out untenable ideas sooner rather than later.

3. Review every investment of time and energy with your partners in the context of your mission and vision, and encourage for and against discussions. Different perspectives may highlight weaknesses not foreseen.

Increasing awareness of project creep across the consortium can build additional capability and competency in managing resources to meet the vision and mission of the consortium while being true to the values that is desires.

Engagement and Motivation

One way to get a handle on motivation is to think of the consortium as a whole person, or an individual personality. At any particular point in time, the consortium can be in a good mood and feel that its work is heading in the right direction. Time passes, events occur, and moods shift into concern, elation, boredom, and so on. Like an individual personality, all of these feelings and thoughts are real and impact performance, interactions, and focus. We get tired, we get energized, we excel beyond our belief, we experience conflict, and we get upset—sometimes, we experience all of these in a relatively short period.

The following ideas can help you minimize and endure the inevitable peaks and valleys of executing a long-term implementation plan:

■   Remember that change is a long journey, one that needs renewal and motivation to avoid burnout. Setting achievable short-term goals can help members experience a motivating sense of accomplishment and see progress toward longer-term goals. Communicate and celebrate these short-term wins.

■   Communicate long-term progress and results on a regular, frequent basis. Over the long term, partners need to see compelling evidence that their journey is producing expected results. Reporting against previously defined measures can help members track progress and provide motivation.

Managing engagement and motivation is a bit like taking the consortium's pulse, documenting symptoms, and responding accordingly. But be proactive in your efforts. Instead of waiting for the consortium to get "sick" before you respond, recognize your members for their work during the up times, too. Recognition not only appreciates your partners' work and motivates to achieve more, but it also makes a statement about the consortium's values. A few guidelines for recognizing your partners' achievements are as follow:

- Develop a recognition plan for noteworthy events and achievements. Clarify the difference between local and regional recognition opportunities; being consistent within the guidelines of the plan allows both local and regional successes to be acknowledged.
- Tie the activity being recognized to the consortium's vision, mission, and values.
- Despite their complexity, large consortia should maintain consistency in the ways they deliver recognition and reinforce the vision, mission, and values.
- Find alternative, fresh ways to recognize the consortium's outcomes and events.

The work of a consortium provides many opportunities to recognize your partners, such as the following:

- Achievement of a goal
- Process improvement
- Creative and innovative solutions
- Partnership accomplishments
- Mentoring and teaching activities
- Professional development activities
- Milestone achievement
- Improved statewide or regional graduation rates
- Improved NCLEX scores
- Successful grant and other funding awards

REPORTING RESULTS AND OUTCOMES

Communicating short-term successes will not maintain motivation and focus in the long run; your members need to see measures of results to stay committed to the consortium's work. One way to track results is through the balanced scorecard mentioned in Chapter 6. If you remember, the balanced scorecard measured four key perspectives of an organization's progress: audience, financial health and stability, process, and people. Table 8.1 suggests outcomes to track and the frequency that they should be reported to meet the needs of the simulation center consortium.

In addition to the key balanced scorecard measures, other process-related measures can provide a good picture of trends and potential correlations. Exhibit 8.2 depicts a few potential process measures for a simulation center consortium.

With the balanced scorecard and other process measures, over time the consortium can begin to evaluate the performance of the total simulation education system and develop trends and correlation of results. Reviewing total consortium performance provides the basis for recognizing individual and team efforts.

TABLE 8.1
An Adapted Balanced Scorecard

DIMENSION	MEASURE	FREQUENCY
Customer	Patient care and safety	Monthly
	Improve critical thinking skills	Per scenario
	Reduce and eliminate medical errors and near misses	Monthly
	CMS measures	Annually
Financial	Actual costs versus budget	Monthly
	Efficiency of process improvement	Monthly
Process	Number of simulation users versus plan	Monthly
	Number of scenarios developed	Monthly
	Strategic evaluation scores	Quarterly
People	Professional development implementation	Quarterly
	Retention rate	Quarterly
	Number of certifications and re-certifications	Monthly
	Evaluation of new hires	Monthly

EXHIBIT 8.2
Potential Process Measures in a
Simulation Center Consortium

- Number of participants at steering committee and task force meetings
- Number of webinar participants
- Meeting newsletter deadlines
- Number of hits on the electronic newsletter
- Number of presentations made to health-related groups on the consortium's vision, mission, and strategy
- Evaluations of webinars by participants
- Number of simulation users participating in online training modules
- Number of attendees at professional development workshops
- Simulation evaluation scores by statement
- Revenue generated across the consortium
- Number of evidence-based scenarios in the library
- Number of participants at open houses
- Status of the project plan and completion of activities
- Success stories and promising practices throughout the region

LESSONS LEARNED

- Provide clear direction by focusing the consortium on its mission and vision.
- Utilize the strengths and resources of the consortium.
- Build capacity ahead of demand.
- Learn from mistakes. They are inevitable and provide valuable learning opportunities.

■ When possible, implement pilot projects to test the impact of activities actions.
■ Communicate rewards and mistakes.
■ Plan resource requirements carefully in advance of action.
■ Create short-term successes to build motivation.
■ Begin thinking of sustainability early in the implementation stage.
■ Provide recognition to reinforce desired behaviors and achievements.

SUMMARY

Executing the strategy is a culmination of a comprehensive planning process that will serve the consortium into the future. With the strategic framework in place, the consortium can carry its business forward with minimal adjustment to the overall direction. The implementation process requires careful attention to goals; managing the various interdependent systems of the consortium, including people, committees, and the flow of work; and preparing for the inevitable challenges. In the future, subsequent strategic planning cycles will run more smoothly and efficiently, and the framework will grow more sound and reliable as the consortium builds upon its successes. A period of renewal and reflection will allow the consortium to learn from its hard work and accomplishments.

SUGGESTED READINGS

Bishop, R. (2011). *Workarounds that work.* New York, NY: McGraw Hill.

Bossidy, L., & Charan, R. (2002). *Execution: The discipline of getting things done.* New York, NY: Crown Business.

Senge, P. M. (2006). *The fifth discipline.* New York, NY: Doubleday/Currency.

NINE

Engaging in Reflection and Renewal

Those who cannot remember the past are condemned to repeat it.
  —George Santayana

The process of building any organizational entity includes not only planning for what will come but also reviewing the strategic activities and goals implemented to identify what went well and what did not (and why the fallout happened that way), find ways to sustain progress, and reconsider or halt initiatives that are not serving the consortium's interests. During the planning and implementation phases, the partners tend to focus tightly on the consortium goals and details of its work. This period of reflection and renewal— taken after the first strategic planning process and first implementation cycle are complete—allows the organization to breathe, take stock, view its accomplishments through a wider lens, reconsider its goals, and develop new, fresh ideas for the future. Throughout the chapter, we will provide guidance, suggest questions, and highlight possible areas for improvement in each step of the simulation consortium model.

WHY SPEND THE TIME?

Breaking the reflection and renewal process into steps that follow the simulation consortium model allows you to organize your conversations and their outcomes. This organization will help you address problems and implement solutions in an efficient and timely way. The process of reflecting on these areas will form the groundwork of the second strategic plan, as well as improve the efficiency of the planning process for several reasons:

1. The time the participants have invested together over the last 1–3 years has created a more efficient collaborative process, as well as a richer understanding of the opportunities for and threats to the consortium's success.
2. The participants see a clearer direction for the consortium, as their understanding of the possibilities of simulation grows. In the beginning, they did not know what they did not know; after 1–3 years, the consortium partners have a much better grasp of their future. As a result, they make decisions more quickly and with greater confidence.
3. The continuous process of planning and action has embedded into the culture and normal workflow of the consortium. No longer a discrete event, planning has integrated into the entire system, which runs more smoothly as a result.

Consortium Development

The consortium has been built, but it continues to develop as an organization. Assess this area in terms of the consortium's assets and liabilities. To ensure that its growth progresses toward a purpose that remains relevant to the consortium partners as well as the nursing profession, consider the following questions:

- Do we have a greater understanding today of the consortium's direction?
- Do our partners exhibit a greater or lesser degree of commitment and engagement since the last strategic plan?
- What concerns do our stakeholders hold?
- What new opportunities or threats have emerged since the last strategic plan?
- What actions have we put in place that need to be continued or expanded?
- What actions do we need to stop or redirect?
- What are the strengths of the various committees?
- How can we leverage those strengths?
- In what areas can we improve? How can the consortium strengthen those areas?

Reviewing and processing the answers to these questions can provide any number of helpful insights, a few of which might include the following:

1. The realization that the consortium leadership has developed somewhat rigid ideas about the organization's needs and how to meet them. Partners may have opinions or concerns about activities or ideas for new approaches. Regional focus groups provide good forums for consortium partners to share their views.
2. New assets and strengths of the consortium have developed over the implementation process. How can the consortium leverage these appropriately?

Measure your consortium's direction against its ultimate destination or goal: If your progress supports and advances simulation education throughout the region, you are on the right track. If not, consider how your strengths can help you change route.

Consortium Leadership and Management

This discussion should evaluate the consortium's roles, structure, vision, mission, and values in the context of the group's greater purpose. The original leadership may no longer provide the best governing structure to carry the consortium forward, and the founding concepts (mission, vision, and values) may no longer reflect the goals of the consortium. Identify the strengths and weaknesses in this area, as well as ways to improve or adapt governing processes, by asking such questions as the following:

- Have the vision, mission, and values changed during the implementation of the strategic plan? If so, is it the result of a healthy scope creep or through inefficiencies and inattention? Has it created confusion or conflict of direction?
- Is the governance structure still appropriate to continue the work of simulation education in the region?
- Are there new opportunities or threats that could influence the direction of simulation education?
- How have the roles of the coordinator and consultant changed over time? Do they continue to serve their original purpose, and does that purpose grow the work of the consortium? Should these positions be removed or changed?

- Should the consortium change its membership to reflect a new environment, players, or emphasis?
- Is funding adequate to continue the regional simulation initiative(s) that are in place or planned?
- What benefits have we seen so far? What new or additional benefits can we expect during the next implementation stage?
- Do the partners experience benefits of implementing the simulation strategy? If not, how can the consortium address that issue?
- How would each partner describe the present consortium environment? What are the norms?
- Is the leadership group engaged and committed to the future direction? If not, how can they increase their motivation?

These questions may highlight several leadership areas to be eliminated, redeveloped, or strengthened, such as the following:

- The vision, mission, and value statements may need careful review, with adjustments to scope and focus, during the next strategic planning cycle.
- The governance structure may require a shift in direction or resource requirements.
- To operate effectively, the steering committee and other governance groups may require new knowledge, skills, and perspectives. Do the current members of these groups educate themselves appropriately, or do the groups take in new members who have the necessary capabilities?
- Funding of the next strategic plan may need to reflect new direction and initiatives, which will impact the consortium's plan for sustainability.
- From the experience of the last implementation cycle, members see the benefits of the simulation initiative more clearly. To reflect this outcome, the consortium may require new and more appropriate goals.
- Because the consortium has finished establishing its working culture, the leadership group may have a better understanding of its strengths and weaknesses.
- The leadership may be better equipped to assess the degree and type of commitment of all partners. How can they increase the motivational level of specific partners? Reviewing those partners' unmet needs may be the first step to take in that effort.

Of course, improving leadership requires good collaborations among consortium members, as well as collaborations among members and the nursing profession. See Exhibit 9.1 for lessons that Debi Sampsel of Wright State University learned about governing structures.

EXHIBIT 9.1
Investing in Committees

Living Laboratory Smart Technology House,
Wright State University
Debi Sampsel

Early on, I did away with a dedicated committee structure because people were finding challenges with time allocation, and I saw it as a burden for them. Committee work is also harder and prolongs the time line—smaller working groups are more efficient, in that sense, but really, it is just a *different* time line. Looking back, I would have kept those committees in place. I think that you get better buy-in when people feel like they own what they are doing rather than advising what you are doing. When you collaborate in committees, you actually contribute to the work, and there is a sense of ownership.

COLLABORATION

Collaboration serves as one of the founding concepts of your consortium, so this review should focus on improving its cooperative systems. By asking the following questions, the consortium can assess collaboration processes to understand how the partners work together and if those processes continue to be successful:

- What have been the specific benefits of working together as a consortium? What actions have led to these benefits?
- What have been the challenges of working together as a consortium? How can these challengers be minimized or eliminated?
- Are we improving in working together, or have we lost momentum?

■ What does our next strategic plan need to improve collaborative efforts?

Reflection upon the answers to these questions will provide information to develop and implement new goals, planning, and other strategies. The consortium might receive such insights as the following:

■ Keeping regular documentation of benefits, challenges, and actions that support collaboration allows you to track the rationale and course of events behind your decisions.

■ We can identify challenges to consortium more clearly with time and experience. Reviewing emerging and unmet needs for simulation centers, and the innovations needed for faculty development and to implement the pedagogy can help realize potential solutions for improvement.

■ A long-standing, complex organization can expect fluctuations in motivation and collaboration. Leaders must learn how to parse real challenges from the natural ebb and flow of commitment, discover their origins, and address them appropriately.

Renewing your members' commitment to collaboration will impact all of your consortium's operations, including strategy development. See Exhibit 9.2 for Scott Engum's thoughts on his consortium's collaborative efforts.

EXHIBIT 9.2
Valuing Input

The Simulation Center at Fairbanks Hall
Scott A. Engum, MD

At the initiation of the building project for the simulation center, the building that we were housed in had already initiated the build-out of the other floors. Our time line was incredibly short to complete all aspects of the project without incurring new construction costs and this did create some pressure on all organizational committee members for timely decisions. Secondarily, the economy was very challenged at the time of the construction, and our governance committee preferred to direct any nonessential funding to patient-related services (a just decision), so we elected to not hire any simulation center staff until we were closer to opening the doors. Our project management company played a critical roll along with the operational committee to fulfill our goals in a timely fashion. Ideally, we understand it is best to have key employees in place at the initiation of planning for such a center; however, the high functioning operational group accomplished all objectives and performed above expectations.

Strategy Development

Reviewing this area of consortium implementation allows you to identify which strategies have worked—and which have not. Your process should rescan the environment to perform a second SWOT analysis that will, in turn, help the consortium develop new core strategies and establish new measures and budgets.

- What does a current analysis of the environment show versus the environment during the first strategic planning process? How have the strengths, weaknesses, threats, and opportunities changed?
- What action items rest in the "reservoir" of possible activities? Which ones are appropriate for the next stage of consortium development? How would you prioritize these items?
- What are the next set of challenges emerging from activities implemented by the consortium?
- Given the members' answers to the previous questions in this section, what are our next strategies?
- Do new measures need to be added to the balanced scorecard?
- What are the budget requirements for the next strategic plan?

The discussion among your partners may provide new discoveries that will affect the priorities and planning for the next several months or so. Potential insights may include the following:

1. The environment identified at the beginning of the first strategic planning process may have changed significantly over the years. As a result, some activities implemented or in the planning stages can be halted.

2. Because the consortium's strengths and weaknesses are products of its makeup, they do not typically change quickly. Opportunities and threats are externally focused and driven, so their rate of development is not entirely within the control of the consortium. The consortium *can*, however, respond appropriately to the environmental factors that impact next strategic plan. The consortium members can also identify those external threats within the community that may require consideration of change or a new direction.

3. A consortium's methods for planning, organizing, directing, and controlling its operations should be much more efficient now. As a result, its members will benefit from more informed decisions in the second and subsequent strategic planning process. The history of the consortium has provided information and data that makes assessments more reliable.

4. Evaluating and addressing potential problems becomes easier because the consortium knows its capability and capacity to create solutions. The consortium becomes more realistic about its resources, strengths, and weaknesses.

5. The reflection process can identify key core strategies to develop, prioritize, and include as the main drivers of action for the next strategic planning cycle.

Because development and assessment work so closely, the consortium cannot refresh its strategic approach without upgrading its evaluation plan.

Strategy Evaluation

The leadership can set the next steps and direction of the consortium by using such questions as the following to assess current strategies:

■ Has the consortium made progress in addressing some evaluation statements to the exclusion of others? Is it appropriate to reprioritize the statements?

■ What new statements could be developed to "raise the bar" of the consortium's performance?

■ If some statements are not viewed as drivers of improvement, can they be removed?

■ If significant progress has been made, how can we recognize the consortium's accomplishments?

■ Have we correlated the evaluation of the strategy against balanced scorecard measures or process measures?

■ Has the leadership shared promising and innovative practices among the regional consortium partners?

Such questions allow the leadership to more accurately assess the consortium's progress and the members' accomplishments. In addition, this process will identify the consortium partners who have been the most successful at meeting their local simulation center goals, as well as those partners who are struggling to do so. By reflecting on the answers to these questions, the consortium members might arrive at the following insights:

■ A strategy for raising the standards in the consortium's areas of success can rejuvenate, motivate, and provide continued excitement and confidence to achieve higher levels of performance.

■ Statements that have not fulfilled their original intent as drivers of excellent performance may be amended or deleted. It is also possible that the statements may not be realistic given the reality of the current environment, and need to be amended or even deleted.

■ Sharing best practices with consortium partners spreads innovation and its benefits. Everyone wins.

■ By analyzing evaluation statements against the balanced scorecard measures and process improvement measures, the consortium can identify and emphasize correlations during the next strategic planning cycle.

Once the strategic plan and evaluation processes are in order, the consortium can begin its review of one of its major strategies: the professional development plan.

Professional Development Plan

Your discussions in this area should focus on the best methods for broadening the scope and depth of knowledge. The consortium needs to ensure that the professional development plan continues to meet the needs of its learners. By nature, the professional development plan fluctuates with the environment, the educational progress of its audience, and changes in technology and pedagogy.

Questions to help you assess your educational scope and adapt the plan as necessary include the following:

■ Has the consortium trained and educated an adequate group of simulation leaders within the region?
■ What emerging topics should be covered in workshops, webinars, online courses, and other professional development opportunities?
■ Does a higher correlation exist between professional development coverage and balanced scorecard measures, or professional development coverage and process improvement measures (especially in patient care and quality)?
■ Do regional libraries or scenario databases contain high-quality content? Do simulation users consider them valuable resources?
■ Are simulation leaders in the consortium being recognized in state-wide, national conferences, research projects, and as presenters in workshops?

After addressing questions like these, the consortium leaders will better understand the professional development committee's level of knowledge and skills in developing, implementing, and evaluating simulations. Based on this information, they might be able to accomplish the following:

■ Identification of a core group of simulation leaders who represent the consortium and work together to train and educate others.
■ Reports of training and education hours or continuing education units for the consortium.
■ An analysis of professional development correlation to key measures.
■ A schedule of funded professional development opportunities for the upcoming year.

Your professional development plan will become more tightly focused and more efficient each year as you apply the lessons you learn through this process. See Exhibit 9.3 for an example of the BASC's lesson on professional development.

Now that the consortium has reviewed its development and planning methods, you can take a hard look at how you have executed your strategy.

EXHIBIT 9.3
Lessons in Scenario Development

BASC
KT Waxman

Interprofessional training has been gaining traction in health care, so our scenarios were written by academic and service partners primarily from nursing. In retrospect, however, I would have partnered earlier with physicians and allied health professionals to develop scenarios. I also learned how to organize collaboration for greater effectiveness. We originally asked groups of 2–4 people to develop scenarios together, but the discussions that ensued just took too long—each person had strong opinions on how the scenarios should be built. Eventually, we streamlined the scenario process so that one person writes the scenario, another subject matter expert validates it, and then another tests it on students. This way, we get different perspectives but equal ownership. The process has become pretty smooth and successful and has generated a solid library of scenarios.

Strategy Implementation

Finally, it is time to review the last stage of consortium development: strategy implementation. Your group should consider if the implementation process has enabled consortium members' growth as well as the achievement of goals. To encourage discussion, consider the following questions:

- What lessons have been learned from the previous strategic planning cycle?
- How can we apply them to the next cycle?
- Do the priorities still remain the same?
- Are there overlaps in implementation? Is there a more efficient way to implement in a collaborative method, e.g., scenario development and review?

The consortium can use the discussion to decide upon improvements to the next strategic plan. Possible ideas for improvement include the following:

- Group insights into categories with similar characteristics or themes. This activity focuses the key lessons learned versus dealing with a multitude of ideas that may take more energy to resolve than is necessary.
- Determine how lessons learned can be applied into the next planning cycle. For example, one consortium had successfully involved partners in simulation scenario development; however, the staff support team did not realize that they had underestimated the partners' capacity to take on more responsibility. Once this information was shared among the group, it was able to identify and implement additional process improvement ideas.
- Continued monitoring of the balanced scorecard and process measures to see the impact of actions on outcomes.

At the end of this process, the consortium should have identified lessons that the consortium can apply in the next implementation cycle.

LESSONS LEARNED

- Documenting the work of the consortium as you proceed pays dividends in times of reflection and renewal.
- Recalling assumptions and motivations behind actions and coupling that information with results and outcomes in the balanced scorecard allows you to learn from your actions. The value of the process is being able to apply your lessons to the next cycle of planning and implementation.
- Over time, the strategic planning framework becomes easier to understand and use. The array of tools, techniques, and processes begins to form a predictable linkage of actions that become more increasingly productive. Eventually, this framework will support your thought processes about large and complex simulation projects.

■ Strategic planning for the next cycle is much faster and easier to perform. You will notice that, in retrospect, the consortium has been planning and implementing its ideas as part of a continuous process.

SUMMARY

Throughout the book, we have aimed to provide a framework of continuous planning and integrated actions that will lead to continuous improvement in simulation education and application. Hopefully, the questions and suggested insights throughout this chapter will help your consortium review your organization's progress and discuss necessary changes to ensure your organization's continued growth. Reviewing and analyzing both successes and failures enable consortia to renew their commitment and refresh their approaches toward the goals of simulation education advancement.

REFERENCES

Santayana, G. (1905). *The life of reason; or, the phases of human progress* (Vol. 1). New York, NY: C. Scribner's Sons.

Juran, J. M. (1989). *Juran on leadership for quality: An executive handbook.* New York, NY: The Free Press.

Planning for Sustainability

Happiness belongs to the self-sufficient.
   —Aristotle

W hat do the following situations have in common?

- A young woman starts her own business.
- A couple in their early 60s considers retirement.
- A consortium with a simulation center project completes the implementation of its first strategic plan.

A hint: Here are some questions that each is asking:

- Do enough assets (benefits) exist to fund this effort, and if so, at what level of expectations?
- What are the costs of this effort, and at what level of expectations?
- What factors are involved in continuing this effort, and at what level of expectations?
- What options are available to either increase assets (benefits) or decrease costs and level of expectations?
- What is the right decision, and when should it be made?

The situations and the questions all have a central theme: sustainability!

Strategic planning sustains the benefits of each subsequent planning cycle and execution. A consortium should address the issue of sustainability at least a year before the end of the strategic planning process. Doing so will provide enough time to develop a plan for sustainability and begin its implementation. This chapter will review information to help consortia accomplish the following:

- Identify the benefits of simulation within the consortium
- Analyze the key factors to sustain the projects

■ Develop a sustainability plan
■ Explore funding options

SUSTAINABILITY AND BENEFITS

The Center for Civic Partnerships (2001) defines *sustainability* as the continuation of a program's benefits. A sustainable consortium, then, manages and builds the benefits of simulation education throughout the region. Such benefits include the following:

■ Improving safety and patient care
■ Improving critical thinking skills
■ Reducing transition time for new graduates
■ Increasing confidence and competence of simulation participants
■ Reducing and eliminating errors and near misses
■ Improving retention rates
■ Improving staff communication
■ Reducing costs of the overall health care system, e.g., shorter stays, more accurate diagnosis
■ Improving efficiency through process improvements
■ Reducing liability costs
■ Encouraging interdisciplinary teamwork

Your consortium may not experience all of these sustainability benefits, but to measure the success of your plan, you will want to identify those most important to your consortium by reviewing the consortium's early simulation research, balanced scorecard, and process measures, as well as consulting your consortium members. (See Exhibit 10.1 for the OSA's ideas on how to take your consortium's sustainability temperature.)

For us, sustainability also means building and sharing our body of knowledge. We have taken our model and adapted it to meet the needs of other consortiums, such as the BASC and the Mississippi Simulation Alliance. We help other consortiums frame their picture of success—what success looks like to them. A lot of organizations do not do that upfront, so they lose focus during implementation. Sharing what we have learned is a win-win situation: It allows us to understand the market and identify the players in a broader sense, which provides perspective on the OSA's audience and goals, and it allows the state or region we are working with to adopt a strategy that

---

EXHIBIT 10.1
Sustainability Requires Flexibility

Oregon Simulation Alliance
Michael Seropian, MD, and Bonnie Driggers

Revisit your goals regularly. Check that you are on course with your mission, and identify any threats. Ask yourselves: Why do we exist? Should we continue, and if so, how so? Are we serving the purpose for which we were created? How should we react to new factors?

---

makes sense for their environment. It cannot be a one-size-fits-all approach.

Your initial literature search should identify benefits, challenges, and current practices of simulation education. The consortium will probably not have realized all of those benefits, but a comparison between them and the benefits that the consortium's current strategic plan highlights will help you spot those valued most by your members. You can also review benefits detailed through the balanced scorecard and process measures developed during the strategic plan process.

You can also interview simulation users and steering committee members. Focus group meetings can also yield additional information. As cycles of planning and action occur, you will see the number and type of benefits increase significantly.

Key Factors of a Sustainable Simulation Consortium

To continue to provide benefits, a simulation consortium must meet several key requirements of sustainability, as follows:

1. It meets the simulation needs of the region, state, or the designated area.

   During its early stages, a simulation consortium conducts a needs assessment that identifies problems in the current state of nursing education, how simulation technology can address those problems, and how a consortium can provide simulation technology and learning resources to educate nursing students and professionals across the region. The consortium fine-tunes the assessment by gathering information on the user audience as well as the assets of the region and begins to shape a flexible strategy to meet user needs.

2. A committed core leadership group is in place.

The commitment of steering committee members and simulation leaders is critical to formulating the strategic plan and carrying its implementation forward. The initial structure of governance and development of an aligned strategic plan assures that projects are aligned with goals that the consortium wants to achieve.

3. Additional stakeholders are enrolled and motivated to participate.

Other groups or organizations that have similar missions are drawn into the consortium as partners and/or interested parties. Not only do they see the benefits of the consortium's vision and mission, but also their own organizational needs for education and training are being met. As this group joins together, the assets available to the entire consortium increase through joint projects, sharing of resources, and generation of new ideas and benefits.

4. The consortium builds positive relationships and identifies joint assets.

As the consortium develops its strategic plan, it also establishes a budget that is funded through a variety of sources, such as membership fees, grants, fee for services, internal self-funding, and in-kind service. With an increasing stakeholder base, the assets continue to grow. Partners also enjoy a wider pool of resources to identify and access funding options. Rather than inadvertently creating financial waste, consortia can use funding more effectively to increase simulation's benefits among the partners.

5. The consortium demonstrates that it produces positive results with the assets it has available.

The balanced scorecard and process measures provide regular feedback on progress against performance goals. Results enhance sustainability when they demonstrate that the consortium's actions meet key goals. A strong communications system allows both stakeholders and the public to see consortium outcomes. The strategic planning process has built an infrastructure that reinforces and promotes positive results throughout the region.

6. A succession plan for key leadership positions ensures successful transition of the consortium's work into the future.

    Training and development of future simulation and community leaders is our best method to ensure sustainability. The professional development plan provides opportunities for knowledge and skill acquisition on a regular basis. An analysis of regional performance against the education and training matrix can track progress and identify areas for improvement.

    The transition of leadership and succession plans are key elements of subsequent planning and implementation cycles. These key elements cannot be left to chance.

DEVELOPING A SUSTAINABILITY PLAN

A consortium may find it difficult to adequately address the issue of sustainability until the benefits of simulation education have been experienced and documented throughout the consortium. Therefore, the initial strategic plan needs enough funding and resources to provide financial security to get through the implementation period, which can run from 8 to 32 months.

Once a measure of success has been achieved, the consortium can begin to address the issue of sustainability much more concretely: Stakeholders have solid data supporting the benefits of investing in simulation to both their organizations and the entire region. At this point, the consortium needs to develop a clear picture of current and future activities that will maintain or increase these benefits.

Begin by reviewing the implementation plan to identify and organize those key activities that lead to benefits. Some will be one-time activities that helped create the infrastructure, such as the creation of a regional scenario library, so you will not consider these as part of the sustainability plan (although the maintenance of the library *is* sustainable). If some implementation activities were not as effective as hoped, eliminate these from future plans; other activities, such as IT support, management of the scenario development processes, and reporting of simulation usage and shared practices, can be transferred and shared by other organizations and partners before the next planning cycle. Finally, note new activities that have resulted from earlier activities. For example, some consortia have reported that conducting simulation facility tours with other educators has increased the number of simulation activities implemented within the institution. Other consortia have also reported that community group tours of the simulation facilities increase their awareness of simulation's positive impact on the quality of patient care. As a result, some civic groups have offered to help fund certain applications that they find important to their organization. Such changes work to continue or expand the benefits of simulation. The combination of these activities—those activities from the strategic plan that are eliminated, transferred to others, maintained, and new—make up the sustainable activities for the next strategic plan. See Exhibit 10.2 for simulation education benefits experienced by one consortium.

Armed with a good understanding of the benefits of simulation, the activities currently supporting them, and activities that might produce benefits in the future, the consortium can begin to form a sustainability committee to gather input from regional partners on the sustainability plan. These discussions shed light on the

---

EXHIBIT 10.2
Simulation: Means to an End

Southeastern Indiana Health Care Consortium
Dave Galle

Moving simulation into administrative process improvement will be a good way for us to sustain the benefits of simulation across an organization. It will allow the administration to see simulation as a means to an end—rather than an end in itself.

More and more locations are melding simulation into the way that they work—one hospital announced that all new processes will be simulated, filmed, and presented so that employees can talk through the flow. Simulation continues to grow beyond to process improvement. Locations look at operating rooms, interactions between doctors and nurses, using simulation with families for home care. Simulation has taken off if directions we would never have predicted. We are truly limited only by our imagination.

benefits that each partner perceives and identifies the activity that contributed to them. After several such meetings, the structure of the sustainability plan begins to take shape. Once the committee has identified all of the beneficial activities, it can begin targeting the resource requirements for sustainability.

FUNDING OPTIONS

Funding, clearly, plays a major role in developing the sustainability plan. Possible resources include the following:

- Cash contributions
- Membership fees
- Federal, state, and local grants
- Foundation grants
- Cost reduction of internal process improvements resulting from simulation education
- Support from community organizations
- In-kind donations or service
- Fees for service
- Endowments
- Leverage of resources among partners

Identifying appropriate sources requires time, energy, and research, so you will need to build this work into your sustainability plan, along with defining benefits, clarifying future strategies for sustainability, building relationships with potential funders, and developing funding strategies. Debi Sampsel of the Living Laboratory Smart Technology House, which is a part of the Nursing Institute located at Wright State University, addressed these issues in part by expanding the educational mode. She has tapped MBA students to examine the Living Laboratory's sustainability plan and marketing feasibility, noting that "we can't sustain ourselves in a volatile economy through only donations and grant monies, therefore, we had to look at the business side of simulation." Our business development has included advice from many business owners, as well as state and federal business organizations. (See Exhibit 10.3 for more information on Wright State University's sustainability plans.)

EXHIBIT 10.3
Generating Income for Sustainability

Wright State University, Living Laboratory
Debi Sampsel

We are evaluating different avenues to generate income for sustainability. We have experienced two financial stability phases of a four-phase business plan. Our first phase, which is now closed, accepted funding from HRSA and the Department of Education. In the second phase, a total quality management accountability system drives the sustainability payment of funding. It includes organizations that have invested operational funding and provided oversight through a sustainability board. We use the monies to generate research and develop projects, some of which will evolve into sellable products. The product sales are projected to generate operational replacement funds.

In phase three, we hope to leverage the product sales while adding new sustainability partners. This approach will help us become more self-reliant. Phase three will be challenging, as we are poised to make a decision to become a not-for-profit company or remain a consortium that is fiduciarily managed by Wright State University.

Phase four of our business plan is total sustainability. The various initiatives need to net enough cash to pay for the direct and indirect operational costs and create a reserve fund on which to draw. We will sustain ourselves through generated income, grants, and replicating services offered in different marketplaces. For instance, our operational funds can help us bridge periods of low usage in the simulation laboratory.

We have woven our work with remote presence telehealth robotics into our simulation education and care delivery research as a new approach to generating self-sustaining funding. We are also exploring the development of commercial products through partnerships with existing companies, such as the use of existing voice activation commanding processes with simulators. A market feasibility study of this potential product has been completed. Selling of licenses for this product would generate income for continued research, development, and operational stability.

An integrated, ongoing, and blended process of these activities built on the consortium's vision, mission, and strategies ensures that the organization targets funding sources wisely. For a well-considered, creative plan of funding, see Exhibit 10.4.

EXHIBIT 10.4
Expanded Funding

BASC
KT Waxman

We are creating a business model for the California Simulation Alliance (CSA) that includes courses, which will bring in some revenue for the CSA. We are now leveraging grant funding from the regional level to seed the CSA, which will become the umbrella organization for all regional efforts in the state. We are moving to a sustainable model with a subscription fee for membership beginning in Spring 2011.

Subscribers will receive a number of benefits, such as fifty free written, validated, and tested scenarios. We have also secured pricing agreements with simulation vendors, so simulation centers, hospitals, and schools will only have access to these discounts if they are subscribers. Eventually, we hope to serve as a virtual entity, a one-stop shop for our subscribers to find best practice models, a network of simulation coordinators, and simulation courses from novice to expert, throughout the state of California. We have five committees established thus far: research, scenario writing, technology, scholarly writing, and policies and procedures.

At the same time, we realize that every region in the state has its own needs and concerns; so ultimately, we want them to be self-sustaining.

Once sustainable activities and funding options have been identified and integrated into the sustainability plan, the committee should review the plan with the steering committee. Upon approval, the plan is ready to be implemented.

CHALLENGES IN DEVELOPING THE SUSTAINABILITY PLAN

No matter how well structured, any sustainability plan confronts challenges. Table 10.1 sets forth many of the common with suggestions to overcome them.

TABLE 10.1
Challenges to the Sustainability Plan

CHALLENGES	HOW TO OVERCOME THEM
The benefits are not clear	Conduct focus group meetings to identify Report against balanced scorecard measures and in-process measures regularly Include success stories in the reporting process Use the communication plan and media to inform others of the benefits
Partners are reluctant to start sustainability planning early enough	Develop a sustainability committee and include sustainability as a regular topic on the agenda of the steering committee
Partners do not agree simulation provides benefits to them	Identify their needs and integrate them into proposed solutions
The consortium places *too* much emphasis on raising money *only*, versus seeking funding that aligns with their vision and mission	Focus on articulating the benefits of simulation education and reaffirming the vision and mission
Funding sources do not understand the consortium's vision and mission or the benefits of simulation education	Strengthen the communications portion of the strategic plan
Individuals do not feel comfortable raising funds	Educate them on the process to build their comfort level Encourage those who are more confident in fundraising to become more active in this role

CHALLENGES	HOW TO OVERCOME THEM
The consortium has not clearly identified a position with fiscal responsibility for new funds and responsibility for implementation	Develop a governance structure and/or memorandum that outlines responsibilities and the decision-making processes

LESSONS LEARNED

■ It is easy NOT to address the issue of sustainability—it is a complex topic that presents many challenges, particularly to consortia that are still establishing themselves; however, almost every one of our consortium contributors mentioned that they wished that they had started planning for sustainability earlier. Do not wait too long!

■ Confront challenges as they arise, so that the consortium can efficiently develop a working sustainability plan.

■ Sustainability can be a creative and energizing process that allows partners to appreciate the benefits of their efforts, as well as combine resources and talents to extend those benefits into the future.

SUMMARY

Although we have identified sustainability as the last element of the strategic planning process, your consortium needs to integrate this activity into the process as early as possible: Without a sustainable, funded set of operations, your consortium can end up spinning its wheels. If built into the system effectively, however, sustainable efforts become a continuous process of integrating planning and action, as seamless as the consortium building model itself.

REFERENCE

Center for Civic Partnerships. (2001). *The center for civic leadership toolkit.* Public Health Institute, Sacramento, CA.

ELEVEN

Evidence of a Successful Consortium

*We shall not cease from exploration, and the end of all our
exploring will be to arrive at where we started and know the
place for the first time.*
    —T.S. Eliot

*I*n this final chapter, we provide not only a summary of the benefits of organizing a consortium using the simulation consortium
model, but a method for assessing the success of your organizational processes. How do we define success? A successful consortium achieves its mission through a long-term series of planning
and implementation cycles that adapt to the needs of its community and provide continuously innovative programs and benefits
to its stakeholders. The PDCA (plan–do–check–act) cycle can help
you visualize that integrative process, and how it leads to success
throughout the simulation consortium model.

THE PDCA MODEL

The PDCA cycle (see Figure 11.1), developed by W. Edwards
Deming in the 1950s (Scherkenbach, 1988), illustrates a continuous
feedback loop that allows organizations to identify sources of variations in programs and products separate from customer or stakeholder requirements.

    In this cycle, each quadrant represents a stage of process
improvement:

- *Plan:* design processes to improve results
- *Do:* implement the plan and measure its performance
- *Check:* assess measures and report results
- *Act:* determine necessary changes to improve the process

Using this cyclic methodology to ensure organizational growth, organizations can achieve success over an extended period. As shown in Table 11.1, the simulation consortium model maps well to the PDCA model.

Together, Figure 11.1 and Table 11.1 show that by following the steps of the model presented in this book, your consortium will continuously improve. When the consortium completes each strategic planning process, executes the plan, evaluates the plan, and reflects on what is learned, it redefines excellence through every PDCA

TABLE 11.1

Comparison of Planning Models

PDCA MODEL	SIMULATION CONSORTIUM MODEL
Plan	Develop the strategic plan Plan for professional development
Do	Implement the strategic plan
Check	Evaluate the strategic plan
Act	Engage in reflection and renewal Ensure sustainability

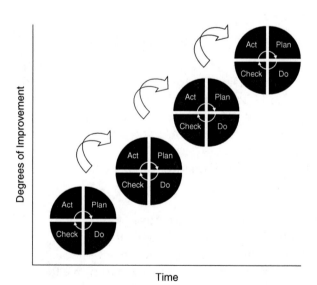

FIGURE 11.1 PDCA cycle.

cycle. Let us see how this cycle helps us evaluate our success as we progress through each of the consortium-building steps.

BUILDING THE CONSORTIUM

Success looks like: The consortium moves toward success when it demonstrates over the course of a planning cycle that it continues to build and retain relationships with key simulation stakeholders. The consortium meets its partners' needs and exceeds their expectations as it identifies and offers innovative programs that use simulation methodology to improve patient care and safety. This success demonstrates that the consortium listens to patient feedback and uses metrics to track improvements in results, such as medical errors, customer satisfaction, incident rates, and other measures of quality. As a result, the regional health care system begins to develop positive referrals and preference—an outcome that provides reinforcement that the strategies and actions put into practices meet patient needs. As these practices improve, health care professionals and educators strive to anticipate future patient needs.

LEADING AND MANAGING THE CONSORTIUM

Success looks like: Regardless of the governance structure, the roles and responsibilities of committees and staff, as well as the reporting relationships between committees and staff, are clearly articulated. The leadership group cooperates in setting the vision, mission, and values of the consortium. The steering committee, along with other working committees, includes representation from each of the partner organizations. Leadership opportunities exist at multiple levels within the consortium, and members exhibit servant leadership in various situations. The consortium culture reflects cooperation, information sharing, and collaboration towards a unified goal.

COLLABORATING WITH OTHERS

Success looks like: Collaboration begins with the consortium's understanding that working together provides greater benefits in achieving their purpose than working alone. Developing partnerships allows each member to learn about and capitalize on the diverse backgrounds, knowledge, skills, and creativity of the consortium members.

Committees and task forces meet regularly and communicate openly and freely. When conflict or differences of opinion present among the group, the consortium provides a forum to discuss the issue, develop options, and implement creative solutions through consensus. Over time, the number of participants in the consortium's problem-solving efforts increases, and as a result, the capacity and capability of the consortium to anticipate and remedy issues do the same.

DEVELOPING THE STRATEGY

Success looks like: A strategic plan has been developed with full participation from the consortium members. The strategic plan includes an analysis of the environment, description of the current state, the future vision, and key strategies to move from the current to the future state. Project goals and objectives have been aligned with strategies and resource requirements to achieve high performance. Leadership ensures that performance measures are clearly articulated and provides regular progress reports. When performance is less than expected, the consortium redirects resources and actions accordingly.

The leadership communicates expectations of high performance and goal achievement to key stakeholders. They recognize staff members, volunteers, and others who achieve those performance levels. Through its work, the consortium reinforces collaboration as a foundational concept and value. Furthermore, the consortium might receive special recognition, and its members were asked to present at conferences. Consortium achievements are publicized through press releases and other media coverage.

EVALUATING THE STRATEGIC PLAN

Success looks like: The strategic plan includes a project plan with a timeline and milestone for each major activity. For each major activity, the planning committee has assigned responsibility and communicated expected results. Resources have been allocated appropriately to support a successful implementation. Individual work plans include goals and objectives that are aligned with the overall strategy of the consortium.

Such process measures as a balanced scorecard evaluate short- and long-term results from different perspectives. Additional in-process measures confirm that processes and programs provide results that support the balanced scorecard measures.

The leadership group reviews performance on a regular basis and provides an environment that values both accountability and cooperation. Staff members feel that they have the resources and support to achieve their goals, as well as the freedom to apply their own initiative and creativity in determining how end results are achieved. As a learning organization, the consortium values mistakes as learning tools, applying these lessons in future decisions and activities.

On a broad and long-term basis, the consortium develops a set of comprehensive evaluation statements that assess all sections of the strategic planning process. Because the consortium values continuous improvement, it ensures that evaluation statements are reviewed and updated on an annual basis to help shape future strategic planning cycles, goals, and objectives.

Most importantly, regional stakeholders see evidence that simulation has made a major impact and difference in achieving patient care and safety goals, as well as other key customer-focused outcomes.

PLANNING FOR PROFESSIONAL DEVELOPMENT

Success looks like: The consortium integrates learning into its operations by

- considering it a daily activity;
- practicing it at personal and organizational levels;
- recognizing its value in solving problems;
- building and sharing knowledge throughout the organization;
- using it to affect significant and meaningful change.

Engaging members in their own learning reinforces the values of the consortium and expands its commitment to education. A successful consortium offers a variety of learning opportunities to address multiple learning styles and increase workforce capability and capacity, including knowledge, skills, and competencies. Measures evaluate the efficiency and effectiveness of learning and development modules. Evidence shows that learning is shared throughout the region in a systematic fashion that is accessible to all members.

IMPLEMENTING THE STRATEGY

Success looks like: Executing a consortium's strategy requires a variety of responses by both leaders and members, including the patience and willingness to let work processes play themselves out, learning to anticipate and manage obstacles and solve problems through the implementation period, and experiencing the satisfaction of seeing actions translate into positive results that are aligned with the consortium's mission and strategy.

While the partners recognize that today's solutions are the sources of tomorrow's problems, they also know that this process is simply part of the development cycle. They also know that by increasing their problem-solving abilities, tomorrow's problems will provide opportunities to use their creative knowledge, skills, and abilities toward greater overall improvement. This cycle eventually becomes integrated into the consortium system, because the measured performance results reflect progress in achieving the consortium's mission.

ENGAGING IN REFLECTION AND RENEWAL

Success looks like: Upon completion of the first strategic planning and implementation cycle, the consortium should take time to reflect on lessons learned. Good documentation through the implementation cycle will provide many ideas for improving the next cycle. The consortium can benefit from these insights by integrating them into the next strategic plan. Reflection and renewal reinforce the consortium's identity as a learning organization and enable it to maintain momentum through future cycles of success.

ENSURING SUSTAINABILITY

Success looks like: A sustainability plan is put into place at least 1 year before it is necessary. The plan describes the governance structure, the benefits to be sustained, and the resources needed to sustain them. The steering committee directs the development of the sustainability plan, often with the help of a sustainability plan committee. These leaders often serve as key fundraisers, since they typically have positional power within their organizations. Their business network with other key stakeholders makes them an invaluable resource in raising the level of interest and funds needed to sustain success. For a look at one consortium's version of sustainability, see Exhibit 11.1.

EXHIBIT 11.1
A Self-Sustaining Business Model

BASC
KT Waxman

The BASC's umbrella organization, the CSA, has had no direct funding, so it has always been the goal to move the CSA to a sustainable business model. We have provided the following benefits to our 3,000 "members" (simulation users across the state) since 2007:

- Savings of more than $1.5 million within the BASC in equipment purchases
- Access to statewide pricing agreement with Laerdal Medical
- More than 50 scenarios developed and available for sharing (over 1,000 scenarios have been distributed to over 300 organizations)
- Statewide simulation survey
- List of simulation coordinators in the state
- More than 40 classes
- Training for more than 1,000 faculty, representing 60% schools and 40% hospitals
- Magic in Teaching (MIT) conference
- Consulting services for each of the seven regional collaboratives
- Bimonthly newsletters

Leveraging funding from both the Gordon and Betty Moore Foundation and from the Kaiser Permanente Community Benefits Program, we have been able to offer monthly simulation training classes throughout the state. More than 15 trainers have emerged from our program, and we have been asked to provide training and consulting services to areas outside of the state. These courses, scenarios, and consulting services are now CSA "products," which will be leveraged for our sustainability.

THE CONCEPT OF CONTINUOUS IMPROVEMENT

In our experience, "continuous improvement" is precisely that; progress that moves forward indefinitely. This concept motivates organizations to continue to achieve and expand their missions to meet the needs of their audience. The PDCA cycle illustrates this never-ending circle of planning, implementation, and improvement in the symbiotic relationship between consortia and the communities they support. Problems and obstacles inspire new hopes, knowledge, skills, and innovative applications to continuously improve the organization's mission, vision, and work. The cycle is endlessly energizing because it allows and encourages growth, commitment to education and community, and self-reflection.

REFERENCE

Scherkenbach, W. W. (1988). *The Deming route to quality and productivity: Road maps and roadblocks*. Washington, DC: CEEP Press Books.

SUGGESTED READINGS

Imai, M. (1986). *Kaizen*. New York, NY: Random House.

Pfeffer, J., & Sutton, R. I. (2000). *The knowing-doing gap: How smart companies turn knowledge into action*. Boston, MA: Harvard Business School Press.

Index